THE URIC ACID HANDBOOK

A Beginner's Guide to Overcoming Hyperuricemia

URVASHI GUHA & SOUMITRA SEN

ULYSSES PRESS

Published by:
ULYSSES PRESS
PO Box 3440
Berkeley, CA 94703
www.ulyssespress.com

ISBN: 978-1-64604-463-4
Library of Congress Control Number: 2022944085

Printed in the United States
10 9 8 7 6 5 4 3 2

Acquisitions editor: Kierra Sondereker
Managing editor: Claire Chun
Editor: Renee Rutledge
Proofreader: Barbara Schultz
Front cover design: Rebecca Lown
Layout: Winnie Liu
Interior artwork: page 23 © Ali DM/shutterstock.com

NOTE TO READERS: This book has been written and published strictly for informational and educational purposes. It is not intended to serve as medical advice or to be any form of medical treatment. You should always consult your physician before altering or changing any aspect of your medical treatment and/or undertaking a diet regimen. Do not stop or change any prescription medications without the guidance and advice of your physician. Any use of the information in this book is made on the reader's good judgment after consulting with his or her physician and is the reader's sole responsibility. This book is not intended to diagnose or treat any medical condition and is not a substitute for a physician. This book is independently authored and published and no sponsorship or endorsement of this book by, and no affiliation with, any trademarked brands or other products mentioned within is claimed or suggested. All trademarks that appear in ingredient lists and elsewhere in this book belong to their respective owners and are used here for informational purposes only. The authors and publisher encourage readers to patronize the brands mentioned in this book.

CONTENTS

STAN'S JOURNEY WITH URIC ACID

Stan was a 1990s Stanford graduate in pharmaceutical sciences. With an interest in communications, pursuing a career in health-care advertising seemed like a great option for him. Eventually, Stan got through campus placements and landed an interview at the firm Sanofi, which hired him on the spot. Still, his heart was in the campaigns run by QR Associates, another health-care advertising firm that aligned with his values around life balance and flexible scheduling. At an award gathering, Stan got the opportunity to meet the CEO of QR Associates. Though many years Stan's senior, the CEO shared his professional interests and immediately took to Stan. They exchanged contact information and kept in touch periodically. The year flew past, and Stan busied himself as part of the brand management team at Sanofi. He soon fell in love with Debbie, a coworker on the Sanofi team. One thing led to the other, and they moved into an airy apartment overlooking the Bronx, a few miles away from the hustle and bustle of Madison Avenue.

One busy morning, Stan was surprised to get a call from the QR Associates CEO, who made him an offer, and his career zipped forward. With dedication and stellar client management, he climbed the corporate ladder quickly. Feeling settled, he proposed to Debbie, who was over the moon to accept, and they got married.

Stan, always at the top of his game, developed quite a business reputation, and big-name clients swooned over his leadership abilities. His office wall was adorned with many trophies and medallions. On the personal front, Stan and Debbie were expecting the arrival of a baby girl. At 40, Stan gloated over the luck of having the best life New York could offer.

But slowly, what began as a small irritant began snowballing into a larger, looming issue. Running was second nature to Stan. A crucial part of his morning, taking a run was a time he took for himself, when he listened to music or podcasts, replayed ideas, played out briefs that his team had received from clients, or made plans for the day. This was his way of remaining a step ahead in life.

But, lately, Stan had begun to feel a bit heavy in his left foot while running. On one run, he even had trouble walking. It was initially annoying, something he considered a minor inconvenience that he didn't want to give in to. He stayed away from running for a week and seemed to have found some relief. Believing he had gotten over the dragging-left-foot problem, he began running again.

When he stepped out for a run again, annoyingly, that feeling of heaviness in his left leg returned as he finished his first mile. It had grown even more painful. Stan could barely keep the quick pace he was used to. He gradually slowed down, and after a while, when he could take no more, he began dragging his left foot again. He was expecting a busy schedule in the upcoming days, and this cursed left foot would spoil everything.

Stan limped back home, took a quick shower, and tried desperately to keep his exasperating left foot out of his thoughts. Debbie waited patiently at the breakfast table as he prepared for the office. The condition of his foot was gnawing at him, so he decided that it was about time that he discussed it with Debbie.

Stan arrived at the table trying to look positive and happy. He gave Debbie a warm hug and a kiss. After clearing his throat, sipping his coffee, and checking his messages, he nonchalantly dropped the news of his problem with his left foot. Debbie listened intently, thinking about what could be responsible for Stan's injured left foot

THE URIC ACID HANDBOOK

over the past month and a half. After a few moments of thought, Debbie attributed the entire problem to Stan's running. Debbie believed Stan was suffering from plantar fasciitis, a condition typical to runners, where the ligaments on the bottom of the feet become inflamed and often cause heel pain. Debbie told Stan that she would read up on plantar fasciitis.

As Stan headed to the office, the words "plantar fasciitis" kept ringing in his mind. *Why didn't it occur to me before?* he asked himself.

In his office, he searched for YouTube videos explaining simple exercises to tackle and manage the issue. Stan wanted to begin them immediately, but he received an email from his boss, inviting him to present a paper in Barcelona for a global conference next week.

Stan had many things to do before Barcelona. This would be his first opportunity to meet representatives from different countries. And, of course, he was looking forward to the exotic food and local alcohol. It also presented the perfect time to take a break from running, rest his feet, and concentrate on the conference. On the way home, he stopped at a pharmacy to pick up some ibuprofen. Stan made up his mind to take ibuprofen twice daily after meals and regularly do YouTube exercises to help relieve the inflammation in his foot.

For the next few days, Stan stopped his morning jogs altogether and began his self-prescribed medication and exercises as he prepared to fly to Barcelona. Stan started to feel the effects of the anti-inflammatory drug almost immediately.

On the day of his flight, the pain in Stan's left foot returned slightly, though not to its former intensity. He found the walk from the airport entrance to the boarding gate quite bothersome. But seated in business class, Stan soon forgot about his foot, as the possibility of meeting new people built up his excitement of visiting a city known for its incredible architecture. His happy and energetic boss kept him company throughout the flight, and Stan used the time on the comfortable flight to go over his presentation and take a restful nap.

As soon as Stan stepped out of the airport, the pain in his foot returned. It soon became challenging to keep pace with his boss as they moved through customs and waited for their luggage to arrive. Walking to the taxi, Stan dragged his feet and silently thanked his stars that his boss was too engrossed in his travel and itinerary to notice Stan's struggle to keep up.

The conference began early the next day. By now, Stan was in considerable pain and seriously worried about his troublesome foot. As everyone retired to their rooms in the evening, they decided to meet in the hotel lobby and walk to the famous boulevard of La Rambla. Stan dreaded such an excursion but didn't want to back out of it and drove away his weariness.

Stan shared his taxi with Dr. Rajendran, the office head from New Delhi, India, with whom Stan had an easygoing conversation on the short ride.

Unbeknownst to everyone in the group, once Stan stepped out of the cab and began walking to La Rambla, Stan was trying desperately to keep up. His tall, athletic frame gave him the aura of a confident man. His struggle, however, didn't escape the notice of Dr. Rajendran, who ran a clinic in the evening after leading the QR Associates office during the day.

Dr. Rajendran subtly invited Stan to step into a nearby café, where he broke the ice without much ado and asked Stan about his foot. Stan knew Dr. Rajendran's reputation as a clinician, so he sheepishly told him that he thought he was suffering from plantar fasciitis, including details of the festering pain, his hectic lifestyle, and how difficulty coping. He added his theory that the pain was probably a result of him overexercising his feet during his runs. Dr. Rajendran considered all this but ended up disagreeing. He shocked Stan by telling him that he suspected Stan was suffering from an acute gout attack caused by high levels of uric acid in his blood, that it required a clinician consultation on his return.

Dr. Rajendran suggested that Stan immediately stop exerting his feet as much as possible until he could meet with a doctor, get the required tests, understand more about his condition, and start taking the proper medications along with rehabilitation as guided by his clinician and team.

Stan listened to Dr. Rajendran in stunned silence, but his pharmacy and health-care communication background told him this could be the case. He was now forced to consider that what ailed him wasn't plantar fasciitis, but gout and high levels of uric acid. *Why did I delay a visit to the doctor?* he thought to himself.

Stan and Dr. Rajendran discussed what could be done to alleviate his suffering. Both men knew that modern science has time-tested drugs to tackle and manage the condition successfully. However, Stan worried that this the condition could prevent him from keeping to his current active lifestyle. After meeting with both his boss and Dr. Rajendran, Stan cut short his trip and flew back home to give his ailment immediate attention.

On the plane, he called Debbie and told her about Dr. Rajendran's his clinical deduction. She volunteered to arrange a doctor's appointment for Stan when he returned. With her health-care background, Debbie knew that he would have to undergo some tests to conclude that he had gout.

Stan thought about how his life had led him to possibly having gout. His lifestyle had been going a bit over the top the past few years as parties with clients and colleagues had become routine. He knew that food containing purines (a compound that leads to the creation of uric acid in the body), like red meat, seafood, and alcohol are prime reasons for high uric acid levels, which can result in gout. Stan tried to think of the last time he visited a doctor, and nothing flashed in his memory of recent years. He quietly confronted this reality and decided to start a lifestyle adjustment the moment he returned home.

The day after returning home, Stan walked into the office of Dr. O'Reilly, his primary care physician. Stan then underwent a quick checkup, blood test, x-ray of his foot, and ultrasound. Although the blood report would take about a day to come back from the lab, Dr. O'Reilly told Stan that, in his experience, this was gout. Dr. O'Reilly wrote him a prescription for treatment with Zyloprim, an allopurinol medication to reduce high levels of uric acid in the blood. The doctor advised Stan to take 100 mg once daily for the first week, then increase the dosage to 200 mg in the second week, and then to 300 mg in the third.

Stan scheduled another visit for a month later, and Dr. O'Reilly assured him that he would feel much more comfortable with his foot by then. To tackle the pain in the meantime, Dr. O'Reilly also prescribed a prescription brand painkiller. They also discussed dietary changes and other lifestyle adjustments needed to keep his gout in check. Stan would need to take nutritional supplements like alpha lipoic acid (ALA) and different vitamins like B1, B6, and B12. Stan expected the reports to confirm vitamin deficiencies, which is generally the case with people suffering from gout. As he shut his phone off and was about to drive away, he received a message from Dr. O'Reilly's staff asking him to visit the nutritionist at the doctor's office the next day.

Stan felt comforted now as he sped homeward to have dinner with Debbie and her mom. He had already applied for leave from work the following week and was looking forward to a relaxing weekend and the chance to get his health back on track.

*****

Stan's encounter with uric acid is one that many of us face, often without understanding it properly. While everyone's journey is unique, you can see in Stan's story how easy it is for high levels of uric acid to slip into your life and cause health problems you could be unaware of until the pain becomes uncomfortable. Left untreated, high uric acid levels may eventually lead to permanent bone, joint, and tissue damage; kidney disease; and heart disease. It's essential to acknowledge and accept that we may need to change our lifestyles to combat metabolic imbalances like this that drive diseases into our lives.

By picking up this book, you have already taken an important step forward. Insulin resistance, diabetes, fatty liver disease, hypertension, hyperuricemia, cardiovascular disease, stroke, gout, joint pains, obesity and mental health issues have one common enemy: uric Acid.

This book will leave you with an understanding on how small modifications in your mind, body, and soul can change how your body deals with the high levels of uric acid. It will walk you through information on what uric acid is, how it affects the body, and common health risks that are associated with high uric acid levels. The advice, tips, and strategies contained within on ways to manage your uric acid levels and improve overall health can help you or your loved ones to get on with life without uric acid becoming an obstacle.

By the end of this book, you can build actionable steps and a list of recipes, which allow you to eat food that is healthy yet delicious.

CHAPTER 1

DECODING URIC ACID

The story of Stan may resonate with many of us. As we reach middle age or begin to strut toward the lower end of our forties, some of us feel our feet getting heavy and painful. Then, through many hits and misses (presumably more hits than misses), we stumble into our health-care ecosystems, where our physicians inform us that the problem is treatable and this affliction—called gout—is caused by elevated uric acid in our blood. Taking some medicines regularly and making some lifestyle adjustments will most probably take care of the problem. This puts our minds at ease, and we follow the suggested prescriptions and lifestyle adjustments rigorously to quickly return to being our old confident selves. We dive right back into our previous patterns as we begin to feel healthy and normal. Our lives continue as before, and gout and elevated uric acid rear their ugly heads a few years down the line.

It seems safe to say that elevated uric acid and gout are manageable as we are armed and backed with the confidence of our doctors, nutritionists, and the like. Then advancing age brings in other, more critical chronic lifestyle issues like hypertension, elevated blood sugar, or dementia. Our lives become a steady stream of appointments with doctors and hospitals, and the ramifications of elevated uric acid levels take a backseat in the overall scheme of things.

People who are experiencing gout and those who are providing care for it know that gout is a common and complex form of arthritis that can affect anyone. It's characterized by sudden, severe attacks of pain, swelling, redness, and tenderness in one or more joints, most often in the big toe.

But is that all there is to it? What if elevated uric acid levels can cause many other health problems? Here is the surprising bit: Scientific studies have shown that elevated uric acid levels may eventually lead to permanent bone, joint, and tissue damage, kidney disease, and heart disease if left untreated.[1] Research has also shown a link between high uric acid levels and type 2 diabetes, high blood pressure, fatty liver disease, and Alzheimer's disease.

This is the primary reason doctors are now treating elevated uric acid before it can cause any serious problems like gout, kidney disease, or heart disease. They have begun to call this condition hyperuricemia.

What on earth is hyperuricemia?

Hyperuricemia is the general condition when too much uric acid— more than what the kidney is able to filter—is found in the body. This clinical condition can cause crystals of uric acid (or urate) to form, which then settle in the joints, causing gout, which can be very painful and disrupting. (See Uric Acid Levels on page 20.) These crystals can also settle in the kidneys and form kidney stones, thereby leading to kidney disease.

Hyperuricemia can also lead to a host of diseases and lifestyle disorders and can cause problems in day-to-day functioning. Some examples of them include:

- Obesity
- Diabetes
- Chronic kidney disease
- Some forms of cancer
- Rising stress levels leading to high blood pressure
- Psoriasis

---

1 "High Uric Acid Level," Cleveland Clinic, last updated May 15, 2018, my.clevelandclinic.org/health/symptoms/17808-high-uric-acid-level; Haifeng Yu et al., "Relationship Between Serum Uric Acid Level and Nonalcoholic Fatty Liver Disease in Type 2 Diabetes Patients," *Medicine (Baltimore)* 100, no. 33 (2021): e26946, www.ncbi.nlm.nih.gov/pmc/articles/PMC8376353.

The biggest challenge that doctors and researchers are facing is that many among us may be experiencing these health issues without ever linking them to elevated uric acid levels. Doctors may not have a vision of the lifestyle that you lead and until a host of tests are run, it may not be detected that you or your loved ones have an elevated level of uric acid. The scenario becomes more complex when you consider that some people can have high uric acid levels in the body without showing any of the above symptoms.

With all of this in mind, wouldn't you like to keep uric acid in check throughout your life? How about starting early? What advantage would that give you to staying happy, healthy, and well, far into your advancing years? The time has come for us to understand and answer these questions so that we can manage our uric acid levels better and live an enriching life well into our advancing years. The following pages will help you understand the term "uric acid" and its impact on everything to do with being in control of your health.

URIC ACID—$C_5H_4N_4O_3$

Uric acid is a white, tasteless, odorless crystalline product of protein metabolism found in blood and urine. (For the curious-minded, metabolism is the process by which the body changes food and drink into energy. During this process, calories in food and drinks mix with oxygen to make the energy the body needs to maintain life.) Most often, one doesn't think of uric acid unless they are experiencing health issues like kidney stones or gout, but this heterocyclic compound (heterocyclic compounds are organic compounds with a ring structure that contains in the cycle at least one carbon atom and at least one other element, such as N, O, or S) of carbon, hydrogen, nitrogen, and oxygen can be a severe metabolic disruptor in life. As complicated as this scientific structure may sound, uric acid is simply a natural waste product that's created when the body breaks down chemicals called purines. The word "uric" in uric acid, or UA, comes from the fact that it is excreted as a waste product through urine. It usually dissolves in the blood, passes through the kidneys, and leaves the body in the form of urine. More and more scientists and health-care professionals all over the world have started mainstream discussions about uric acid over the last decade given lifestyle changes and the trend of large numbers of people suffering with elevated levels of uric acid.

One question that may now arise is whether uric acid is only a metabolic waste product of the body, with no other use. Nothing can be further from the truth! Uric acid is within us for a reason. This understanding is based on the notion of connectivity. Like everything else in nature, where nothing happens in isolation, a universal connectedness makes life work. So let's try to understand this connectedness in relation to uric acid.

TRAVELING BACK IN TIME

Let's go back a few million years, when our ancestors were very few and their survival was based on foraging for food, mainly fruits. Once a month or every two weeks or so, they scavenged for dead animals killed by predators like tigers, leopards, hyenas, lions, and hunting dogs. With each passing generation, they grew more confident and learned to hunt for the weaker, more vulnerable game whenever the opportunity arose. They were also one of the most vulnerable predators roaming the world foraging, scavenging, hunting, and being hunted.

THE IMPACT OF FRUIT ON PRIMITIVE MAN

What does the history of fruit consumption have to do with uric acid levels in the body? The simple answer is that when the body breaks down fructose, purines are released. As purines are broken down, uric acid is produced. It has been observed that in our body, fructose metabolism can generate uric acid within minutes of fructose being consumed.[2]

To complicate matters further, a gene in the body produces uricase, an enzyme that helps to break down uric acid into the harmless molecules allantoin and ammonia, which are then easily secreted out of the body through the kidney as urine. Had uricase been allowed to secrete uric acid in the blood in an unfettered manner in the bodies of primitive peoples, then uricase would have helped break down uric acid and its levels in the blood would be much lower than those found today. But that is not the case.

In fact, humans have comparatively higher levels of uric acid in the body (see Uric Acid Levels on page 20) compared to fishes and amphibians. This is because the body needs uricase to break down uric acid, but interestingly, increased uricase secretion has been found to interfere with the conversion of fructose into fat. So uricase, which breaks down uric acid, also severely limited the ability of ancient humans to build fat stores from fructose, and therefore, self-limited their ability to break those fat stores to give the energy to live and survive.[3]

So humans evolved in a way that restricted the release of uricase, and then, through several generations of evolution, we managed to completely stop it from releasing uricase altogether. This gene mutation (stopping the uricase releasing gene from working) led to the high levels of uric acid in our bodies today. The overall effect was like turning on a fat switch in our bodies. Foraging for fruits helped primitive people evolve to break down fruits into fat. We learned to conserve our fat stores created by fruit ingestion.

2 Young Hee Rho, Yanyan Zhu, and Hyon K. Choi, "The Epidemiology of Uric Acid and Fructose," Seminars in Nephrology 31, no. 5 (2011): 410–419, DOI: 10.1016/j.semnephrol.2011.08.004.

3 Richard J. Johnson and Peter Andrews, "Ancient Mutation in Apes May Explain Human Obesity and Diabetes," Scientific American, October 1, 2015, https://www.scientificamerican.com/article/ancient-mutation-in-apes-may-explain-human-obesity-and-diabetes.

Fruits provide us with fructose, a type of sugar that, when ingested and broken down, stores itself in the body as fat. These fat stores gave our ancestors energy and helped remove excess sugar from their bloodstream. Over millions of years of evolution, the energy produced from our fat stores gave the ability not only to subsist but also to grow the brain in overall size and complexity to become the biggest expender of energy (almost 80 percent of the energy we produce) in the body.

This, in effect, offered an efficient method for energy storage that ensured less risk of starvation, improving our chances of survival in an unforgiving world.

This gave rise to a situation where there was less uricase in our bodies and therefore more free uric acid in our blood.

This was all okay till we got to eating proteins irregularly; we will discuss this later in the chapter.

EATING MEAT AND ITS EFFECT ON HOMINIDS

Now let's look at scavenging and hunting, far rarer occurrences than foraging for fruits in ancient times. Though scavenging and hunting vulnerable species were rare, our ancestors still stuck to them as doing so provided a source of protein. Proteins help in growing, maintaining, and repairing cells. Excess protein, however, was converted to glycogen, which was stored in the body until the body required it to be further broken down into glucose, which then broke down and became another source of energy. Digesting these animal proteins (in the liver) caused the formation of chemicals known as purines (the ones that formed during the metabolism of fructose or ATP or energy molecules), which was and continues to be an essential process even today. While purines formed and expended energy for our ancestors to survive and forage, uric acid was released as a metabolic end product in quantities that could be easily handled by the body and then excreted as urine by the kidney.

DIGESTION TODAY

It is an interesting moment to pause and consider digestion today. Compared to our ancestors, we modern humans consume excess fructose in the form of fruits and meat daily. We eat more than what is necessary or what the body needs, resulting in our bodies reacting in a manner that may not be advantageous for a healthy lifestyle.

Excess fructose and animal protein are either stored within us as glycogen or converted into extra fat that accumulates over time.[4] All this leads to excess uric acid in the body, which is not easily excreted, and its presence in the body tends to rise to more-than-normal, or elevated, levels (see Uric Acid Levels on page 20). It's important to note here that today our access to fructose and proteins is guaranteed daily, while the primitive peoples could have fruits maybe once in one or two days and protein may be only once every two weeks or even once a month.

Today's excess purine consumption makes it difficult for the body to eliminate excess uric acid from the system, leading to a host of health problems.

The following foods and drinks that are high in purines and can be a factor in raising your uric acid levels today:

- Seafood (especially salmon, shrimp, lobster, and sardines)
- Red meat
- Organ meats, like liver
- Food and drinks with high fructose corn syrup
- Alcohol (especially beer, including nonalcoholic beer)

---

4 Thomas Jensen et al., "Fructose and Sugar: A Major Mediator of Nonalcoholic Fatty Liver Disease," *Journal of Hepatology* 68, no. 5 (2018): 1063–1075, doi: 10.1016/j.jhep.2018.01.019.

A surprising fact to note is that for millions of years, our forefathers lived healthy lives and survived on dangerous terrain without eating carbohydrates. We shall delve more into this in the section Carbohydrates—Necessary or Unnecessary? on page 25. Let's turn our attention back to uric acid. Why is it there in the first place? Do we really need it?

WHY IS URIC ACID IN THE BODY?

Now here is a twist: the body does not just create this metabolic end-product uric acid to throw it out through the kidneys. All the uric acid that is formed because of animal protein metabolism and not destroyed because of a mutated uricase gene has its uses, too.

Our bodies need to maintain uric acid at optimal levels in the blood plasma to ensure that we can stimulate, build, and maintain our immunity.[5] Rotting dead animals and fruits, and changing weather patterns meant that humans needed good immunity to survive the travails of life in a primitive world. Uric acid stepped in admirably to fill stimulate our immunity. This is another crucial result of the mutation of the uricase-releasing gene.

In the scientific community, uric acid is often known as "the immune system stimulant." This is because uric acid has the power to heal scarred tissues in the body by initiating the process of inflammation that is necessary for tissue repair (not all inflammation is bad!). This inflammation helped ancient humans repair open wounds sustained during their foraging and hunting activities and protected them from microbes that often attacked their open wounds. It was and still is a helpful immunological mechanism. As a result, however, it has also

5 Faranak Ghaemi-Oskouie and Yan Shi, "The Role of Uric Acid as an Endogenous Danger Signal in Immunity and Inflammation," Current Rheumatology Reports 13, no. 2 (2011): 160–166, DOI: 10.1007/s11926-011-0162-1.

made us evolve into a mammal that has learned to live with chronic inflammation. Furthermore, as an immune system stimulant, uric acid can eat or scavenge for harmful oxygen free radicals that play truant with various components of the human cell, thus causing their death and destruction. Oxygen free radicals, as we know, are those armies of molecules that can destroy cells. The uric acid that we produce is a key antioxidant in keeping our bodies healthy and fine by checking the proliferation and growth in numbers of these oxygen free radicals.

Another important process where uric acid is produced as a metabolic end-product that helps the body is in the process of cell lysis; i.e., the death of aging cells and maintenance of living cells. Made of millions of cells, the body is constantly in a state of flux. Some cells are aging, some are dying, some are young and robust, and some are just being born. In this wonderful microcosmic world of birth, growth, and death, our uric acid as a metabolic end-product is constantly being released so that we can stimulate, build, and maintain our immunity as each individual cell continues to do the function it created.

URIC ACID LEVELS

Here we present another twist to this exciting tale. Too much or too little of anything is not acceptable. Nature designed everything to be finely balanced. So is the case with uric acid! The levels of uric acid in blood plasma should be in the range of 3.5 to 4.5 mg/dl at the lower level and 7 to 8 milligrams per deciliter (mg/dl) at the highest level for men, and 2.5 to 3.5 mg/dl at the lowest level and 6 to 7 mg/dl at the highest level for women.

A uric acid test can be done as a blood test or a urine test. During a blood test, a health-care professional will take a blood sample from a vein in your arm, using a small needle. After the needle is inserted, a small amount of blood will be collected into a test tube or vial.

LOW URIC ACID LEVELS

The surprising fact is that sometimes uric acid levels in the body go down. These rare occurrences or decreasing uric acid levels, referred to as "hypouricemia," often signal other health problems, like Wilson's disease, which is an inherited disorder that causes copper to build up in the body tissues.

Keeping with our contention that everything in nature needs balance and connectedness, the same rings true for copper. Copper in minute quantities is necessary for health as it works with iron to help form red blood cells. But when it accumulates to a higher level, it may cause brain and liver damage, and even death. Interestingly, a correlation has been found here with uric acid levels. It has been observed that this condition is always accompanied by lower uric acid levels in the body.

Low levels of uric acid also cause a rare kidney disease known as Fanconi syndrome, most commonly caused by cystinosis, where uric acid secretion increases at more-than-normal levels through the kidneys. Cystinosis is a condition characterized by the accumulation of the amino acid cystine (a building block of proteins) within cells. Excess cystine damages cells and often forms crystals that can build up and cause problems in many organs and tissues. Additionally, Fanconi syndrome is often caused due to alcoholism, and this is another reason to keep the habit of tipping the glass in control.

ELEVATED URIC ACID

It is time to focus on elevated uric acid levels, or "hyperuricemia," a more prevalent condition causing various health issues. Let's consider elevated uric acid to mean more than 7 mg/dl for men and 6 mg/dl for women (see Uric Acid Levels on page 20). Anything higher than this signals that someone is heading into a serious zone. The prime manifestation of hyperuricemia is gout, and as mentioned, physicians consider this as the harbinger of other lifestyle disorders like diabetes, cardiovascular issues, liver and kidney disease, Alzheimer's disease, thyroid problems, and erectile dysfunction. Here is an important pointer to note.

It is important to mention here that it is best to describe normal uric acid levels in the body as being in the "Goldilocks zone," which means neither too high nor too low. It's like our lovely blue planet, which is neither too cold nor too hot but just right for life to subsist and persist.

OUR STRONG ANCESTORS AND URIC ACID

Back to our ancient ancestors. Historians, anthropologists, and paleo pathologists have found that our ancestors, before the advent of agriculture some fifteen to twenty thousand years back, sometimes ate only once in two or three days. This kept their bodies and minds in a hyperexcited state of hunger, with their brains urging them to keep foraging for food even after eating a satisfactory stomach-filling meal, as they didn't really know when or where the next meal would come from. Whatever uric acid was being produced due to protein metabolism was used up for stimulating the immune system, and then, that uric acid was further broken down into smaller molecules like allantoin and ammonia, which were easily secreted by the kidneys.

Analysis of human bodies unearthed from this time period has demonstrated conclusively that our ancestors, because of the balanced uric acid levels, always exhibited healthfully low blood pressure compared to modern humans. In fact, research has shown that in those prehistoric humans, there is a lack of association between elevated BP and age, which is something that's taken for granted in our world today. We accept it without any trace of trepidation that blood pressure in our bodies increases with advancing age.

It has been found that our ancestors had far more robust insulin sensitivity and lower fasting insulin concentration in their middle and advanced years than what we find within us today. This meant that diabetes perhaps didn't exist millions of years back. That's not all—our ancestors showed better bone health markers (bone markers are blood and urine tests that detect products of bone remodeling to help determine if the rate of bone resorption and/or formation is abnormally increased, suggesting a potential bone disorder) and lower body mass index (BMI is a measure of body fat based on height and weight that applies to adult men and women), due to the normal levels of uric acid in them.

BMI CHART FOR ADULTS

This graph of BMI categories is based on the World Health Organization data. The different shades of gray, with the lightest indicating underweight and the darkest extremely obese, represent subdivisions within a major categorization.

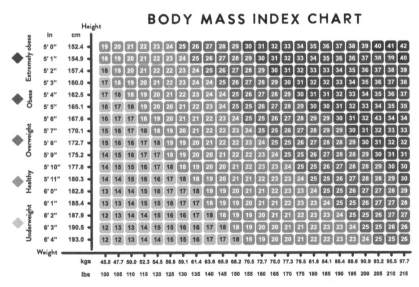

BODY MASS INDEX CHART

Paleo pathologists tell us that our ancestors had less fat, as is evident from lower triceps skin fold measurements from skeletal remains. In fact, they were a far fitter, leaner, and meaner biological machine than the strongest of us today. This means they had more muscle and less fat. You may be glancing at the soft fat layer that has settled so snugly around your stomach while reading these words. Are you? Well, our hunter-gatherer didn't have abdominal fat at all. Whatever he or she ate used to get stored as fat in the body, which was used up immediately by the body as energy in the next two to three days as he or she foraged for more fruits in the wild jungles of yesteryears. Uric acid levels remained normal because animal proteins were ingested rarely, and the little that there was became fat and energy while its metabolic end product uric acid went about fulfilling its positive role in the body. All this makes us conclude that elevated uric acid levels as a health problem was just nonexistent.

HUNGER HORMONES— LEPTIN AND GHRELIN

Early humans regulated the feeling of hunger in a far better manner than we manage to do today. To understand this, it is time to introduce two hormones into our conversation: leptin and ghrelin. A little bit about hormones first. If enzymes like uricase are catalysts of biochemical reactions, reactions that are happening in our body, then hormones are those molecules that act like messenger molecules in the body. After being made in one part of the body, they travel to other parts, where they help control how cells and organs do their work. For example, insulin is a hormone that's made by the beta cells in the pancreas and works in the digestive system to help regulate sugar levels.

The hormone leptin secreted by the brain ensures that we don't feel hungry often, and at the same time, the hormone ghrelin triggers hunger whenever the stomach feels empty. This interplay between leptin and ghrelin ensures that we use our fat stores efficiently and fill our stomachs in a periodic manner. Both these hormones influence satiety and hunger and play a significant role in energy balance and regulation.

You could say that in those ancient times, bodies were programmed to be perennially in starvation mode, and to eat as much as possible whenever possible before the next meal. This gave us the ability to resist the hormone leptin, so the body would not feel satiated, amplifying the effect of ghrelin. In other words, feeling hungry ensured continued foraging for food so there was enough for the next meal.

Today we feel hungry often, do we not? This hunger is often referred to as "hedonistic hunger," which is a hunger that is propelled by the imaginative brain. It makes us imagine a nice fluffy omelette or a rare steak. This makes the hunger juices flow. All this happens because we are programmed to listen to ghrelin and inhibit leptin and its satiety effect. The way we evolved has now come to bite us. Our brains now make us eat more because food is readily available, and foraging or hunting for it is not necessary any longer. The result: we eat more than we need!

Leptin also helps us maintain normal weight on a long-term basis. The level of leptin in the blood is directly related to how much body fat we have, which is directly related to elevated uric acid levels. Leptin resistance causes us to feel hungry and eat more, even when the body has enough fat stores. This leads us to have breakfast, lunch, dinner, supper, high tea, etc., many times in the day. Had leptin levels been high, then we wouldn't feel hungry so often.

CARBOHYDRATES— NECESSARY OR UNNECESSARY?

It's time to solve the carbohydrate puzzle! This brings us to the advent of agriculture. Out of more than three million years on this planet, we spent approximately 2.98 of them ingesting fruits and animal protein. Then, around twenty thousand years back, we discovered and invented agriculture—a big mistake from the uric acid standpoint. Suddenly we added carbohydrates to our diet. Carbohydrates became an abundant food source. Our bodies, which had evolved to eating fruits and berries and animal proteins over millions of years, suddenly began to change their preference without having had the time to adjust. We now consumed the carbs and stored them as fat, which is harder to break down, followed by fructose from fruits and proteins from animals—in that order.

Agriculture gave us an abundance of fruits and animal proteins, too. We grew fruit trees and domesticated animals for proteins whenever we wished. Nature didn't will it that way. With an abundance of carbs, fructose, and proteins, our bodies went haywire. We had already mutated the uricase-releasing gene long before we learned agriculture, as we needed to convert fructose into fat stores. With agriculture, we began to load ourselves with animal protein whenever we wished, daily in many cases, and our bodies began to suffer from an overload of uric acid.

While wanting to become that fitter and leaner, you may also be thinking about how uric acid played a role in making all this happen for our hunter-gatherer friends and suddenly turned to such a villain in its elevated state. Carbohydrates entered the scene and became the dominant nutrient, and with the uricase gene closing shop millions of years back, more fructose got converted to fats and more protein also got converted to fats. As a result, uric acid began to accumulate in our systems, with the body unable to get rid of it all, affecting the BMI. Obesity has become a difficult epidemic to manage and treat.

CHAPTER 2

THE IMPACT
OF DISEASE

By now you have a better understanding of how elevated uric acid causes not only gout but also a host of other medical issues. Consider this for a moment. Nearly half of adults in the United States (47 percent, or 116 million) have hypertension, defined as a systolic blood pressure greater than 130 millimeters of mercury (mmHg) or diastolic blood pressure greater than 80 mmHg, or are taking medication for hypertension.[6] Knowing all this leads us to an important question: Why are rates of high blood pressure (hypertension) going up, even in adolescents and in people who maintain their ideal weight (a staggering one in three adults has hypertension and one in ten youths between the ages of twelve and nineteen has elevated blood pressure)?[7]

Most probably, this epidemic is due to elevated uric acid in the body. According to Peter Grayson MD, a rheumatologist at the Boston Medical Center and lead investigator in a study, most of the studies his team reviewed accounted for factors that are traditionally known to increase the likelihood of developing high blood pressure—such as age, family history, weight, and tobacco use. By doing this, Dr. Grayson and his team were able to determine if uric acid independently increases the risk for hypertension. Among the 18 studies analyzed, there was data from 55,607 participants, including 13,025 participants with high blood pressure. The researchers noted

---

6 "Facts About Hypertension," CDC.gov, last updated July 12, 2022, www.cdc .gov/bloodpressure/facts.htm; See the Centers for Disease Control and Prevention at www.cdc.gov, and the American Heart Association at www.heart.org.

7 "Facts About Hypertension," CDC.gov.

that participants with hyperuricemia were more than 40 percent more likely to later develop high blood pressure than participants without hyperuricemia. Women with the highest uric acid levels and people who develop high levels of uric acid at a relatively young age are especially at risk for developing high blood pressure.

HYPERURICEMIA

The good news is that hyperuricemia can be managed, stopped, and controlled with adequate recognition to asymptomatic hyperuricemia, or elevated uric acid in the body that doesn't exhibit any symptoms. All of us need to add "check uric acid levels" to our health checkup lists. This is because if we let hyperuricemia persist untreated, then its resulting health issues can be severe. The good news is even if we do find out that we have hyperuricemia, it shouldn't be any cause for worry, as it can be fully treated by medication and sustained lifestyle changes.

HYPERURICEMIA AND GOUT

It's now well-known and accepted that the major symptom of hyperuricemia is gout. When uric acid levels are elevated, urate crystals may form stone-like deposits in joints, soft tissues, bones, and skin, and trigger gout flares with episodes of severe pain.

It is important to note that gout is often described as a common and complex form of arthritis with a sudden attack of pain, swelling, redness, and tenderness in the affected location. Without clinical intervention, these urate crystals can become increasingly problematic within affected joints or tissues, and progressively damage them.[8]

---

8 Wei-Zheng Zhang, "Why Does Hyperuricemia Not Necessarily Induce Gout?" *Biomolecules* 11, no. 2 (2021): 280, DOI: 10.3390/biom11020280.

The traditional treatment with uric acid-lowering drugs for gout flares has been well-established for the improvement of quality of life, although it may not be optimal for all patients. Clinicians also employ anti-inflammatory therapy to reduce deposition of urate crystals in the joints. Allopurinol remains the first-line drug for reducing uric acid levels to normal. It is prescribed most often together with colchicine or nonsteroidal anti-inflammatory drugs for enhancement of efficacy.

Drugs like allopurinol and non-steroidal anti-inflammatory drugs (NSAIDs) may not rapidly eliminate local inflammation due to a gout flare. It takes patience and diligence because a full recovery from a gout flare takes time (this varies from patient to patient). This may make a person feel unsure about the regimen that they are following. Here we provide you with a list of drugs used to treat gout:[9]

COMMON MEDICATIONS FOR THE TREATMENTS OF HYPERURICEMIA AND GOUT FLARES

Drug	Brand Name(s)	Therapeutic Function
Allopurinol	Aloprim, Zyloprim	Reduces uric acid production
Febuxostat	Uloric	Reduces uric acid production
Colchicine	Colcrys, Mitigare	Reduces inflammation
Indomethacin	Indocin, Tivorbex	Relieves the pain in the joints caused by gout flares
Probenecid	Probalan	Helps the kidneys excrete uric acid from the body
Losartan	Cozaar	Reduces uric acid levels
Corticosteroids	Orapred, Prelone, etc.	Fights inflammation caused by elevated uric acid

9 National Institute of Diabetes and Digestive and Kidney Diseases, "Gout Medications," *LiverTox: Clinical and Research Information on Drug-Induced Liver Injury* (July 19, 2017), https://www.ncbi.nlm.nih.gov/books/NBK548226.

COMMON MEDICATIONS FOR THE TREATMENTS OF HYPERURICEMIA AND GOUT FLARES

Drug	Brand Name(s)	Therapeutic Function
Fenofibrate	Antara, Fenoglide,	Reduces uric acid levels
Pegloticase	Krystexxa	Breaks down uric acid

An increase in uric acid concentration that exceeds the normal range might not be exclusively linked to gout flares, as many factors causing hyperuricemia are not relevant or significant to gout formation. Certain foods or medicines could induce hyperuricemia. Under renal dysfunction or cell damage, UA could suddenly increase by changing renal function to cause hyperuricemia. Drugs such as diuretics, anticonvulsants (valproate and phenobarbital), cyclosporine, theophylline, favipiravir (an antiviral drug), and pyrazinamide have been reported to increase uric acid levels.

Emotional stress, fasting, or dehydration caused by physical activity can also increase the concentration of UA. Although occasionally, an acute gout flare may be linked with the above-mentioned medication(s) or condition(s), enhanced uric acid levels are generally speaking a temporary phenomenon, and a gout flare is considered unlikely to occur if a longer duration and higher dose treatment are avoided. Controversially, pseudo-gout (a form of arthritis characterized by sudden, painful swelling in one or more of the joints, which can last for days or week), which is caused by calcium pyrophosphate deposition (CPPD), could have the same inflammatory symptoms as gout without hyperuricemia.

NATURAL TREATMENT FOR GOUT FLARES

There are products available that are completely made of natural products, like berries, that help when there is a gout flare. Uric Acid

Complete is one such organic and kosher product that cleanses uric acid from joints naturally. It is a liquid remedy that combines ingredients that are beneficial in helping support kidney function, circulation and the management of uric acid levels.

Such products generally include organic ingredients like water, apple cider vinegar, tart cherry, beet root, lemon, black carrot, peppermint, lime, cinnamon, rosemary, chanca piedra, citric acid, grape, purple corn, red cabbage.

HOMEOPATHY

Homeopathy, also known as homeopathic medicine, is a medical system that was developed in Germany more than 200 years ago. It's based on two unconventional theories:

"Like cures like"—the notion that a disease can be cured by a substance that produces similar symptoms in healthy people.

"Law of minimum dose"—the notion that the lower the dose of the medication, the greater its effectiveness. Many homeopathic products are so diluted that no molecules of the original substance remain.

Homeopathic products come from plants (such as red onion, arnica [mountain herb], poison ivy, belladonna [deadly nightshade], and stinging nettle), minerals (such as white arsenic), or animals (such as crushed whole bees). Treatments are "individualized" or tailored to each person—it's common for different people with the same condition to receive different treatments. Homeopathy uses a different diagnostic system for assigning treatments to individuals and recognizes clinical patterns of signs and symptoms that are different from those of conventional medicine.

Homeopathy treats the root cause of the problem and aims to eradicate the health issue completely. In homeopathy, it is not about controlling the levels of uric acid, but rather ensuring that the levels in the body never go above the recommended range. This means that once you begin therapy for managing your uric acid levels, the homeopathic practitioner works toward getting the levels back to normal and ensures that they stay that way. In homeopathy, increased levels of uric acid is considered a symptom and not a disease, unlike allopathy, which considers hyperuricemia as the main health issue or disease. A homeopath often does a deep investigation to find the reason for elevated uric acid levels in the body.

Homeopathy is known to control uric acid and is also useful in acute attacks. The following drugs can be an essential aid in the treatment of gout if you are keen to follow homeopathic treatment to handle hyperuricemia.

LYCOPODIUM—This drug is used when a patient has:

- chronic gout with chalky deposits in the joints
- mental keenness but shows weak muscular power
- an emaciated (thin and withered) body and tends to have gas
- the feeling of apprehension and fear of being alone
- a lack self-confidence, but a haughty and headstrong temperament when sick
- pain in the heels, as if treading on a pebble
- a hot feeling in one foot but a cold feeling in the other
- urine that is is slow in coming and shows heavy red sediment
- a backache that is relieved by urination
- a right side of the body that is peculiarly affected
- complaints that seem to increase in the evening, especially between 4 p.m. and 8 p.m.

COLCHICUM—This drug has a specific power to relieve a sudden attack of gout but is more beneficial in cases of chronic impact. This medicine is used when the effected parts are:

- red, hot, and swollen with tearing pains felt more in the night
- sensitive to touch
- tearing pains in the joints in hot weather and stinging during cold
- gout that has settled in the great toe or in the heel
- disorders of the stomach accompanying gout
- nausea and even fainting at the smell of food, particularly fish
- an icy coldness felt in the stomach
- urine that is dark, brown, or black, like ink

URTICA URENS—This drug, prepared from the stinging nettle, helps eliminate uric acid from the body. This is used when the patient:

- tends to have gout and stone formations
- has joint symptoms that are associated with urticaria or alternate with it
- has the shoulders (deltoid region), wrists, and ankles affected
- cannot tolerate touch, water, or exposure of the affected parts to cool, moist air and snow air.

LITHIUM CARBONICUM—This drug is used when:

- there is swelling and tenderness of the finger and toe joints, which feels better with hot water
- there is a nodular swelling of the joints
- there is ankle pain on walking
- there are headaches, acidity, nausea, and gnawing pain in the stomach which ceases while eating
- the urine may deposit red sand and is turbid, scanty, and dark
- there are joint symptoms associated with a heart disease

LEDUM—this drug is used when:

- gout is the result of alcoholism
- the inflammation of the joints begins in the lower limbs and ascends upward
- the ball of the great toe is swollen and sometimes red or bluish, and cold to the touch
- dipping the part in a bucket of ice-cold water relieves the pain
- it is generally worse from getting warm in bed
- the patient is sensitive to the cold, yet the heat of the bed is intolerable

BENZOIC ACID—this drug is used when:

- there are symptoms of gout associated with highly colored and offensive urine
- the pains are tearing in the affected joint
- gout seems to settle in the Achilles tendon, just above the heel
- the symptoms worsen in the open air and from uncovering the affected parts

A detailed history followed by constitutional treatment by a qualified homeopathic specialist is necessary to treat gout. It is not advisable to resort to self-medication for any disease. The above-mentioned drugs are just a few of the remedies for gout and are mentioned solely to create awareness about the efficacy of homeopathy in this disease.

AYURVEDIC TREATMENT FOR ELEVATED URIC ACID LEVELS

If you have heard of Ayurveda before and think you would like to give it a try, here are some herbs and remedies from this ancient form of alternative medicine. But first you should know that according to Ayurveda, everyone is composed of the universal energies of five elements: air, fire, water, earth, and space. These elements are present in our system as three doshas: vata, pitta, and kapha.

Vata dosha is related to air and space. When the balance in vata dosha is disturbed, we are prone to stress and anxiety.

Pitta dosha is related to fire and water. It is the energy that helps you digest food and express emotions.

Kapha dosha is related to earth and water. Kapha is considered as the protector; it's the fluid in the joints that softens any shock the body could receive.

These universal energies play an important part in the following methods for healing that help to manage uric acid levels:

1. Punarnava kadha: *Kadha* means "a kind of solution" in Ayurveda. This solution has ingredients like punarnava (*Boerhavia diffusa*, or hogweed), neem (*Azadirachta indica* or Indian lilac), guduchi, kutaki, and daruharidra. It decreases the inflammation that occurs in joints when uric acid is high. Punarnava removes the accumulation of toxins through urination.

2. Gugul: In Ayurveda, it is considered a painkiller as it reduces pain and inflammation around the joints, and helps in controlling uric acid levels.

3. Guduchi: This is the main drug of action for uric acid. It reduces the pitta amount. It helps balance pitta and vata dosha and decrease uric acid in blood. It also relieves pain and inflammation of the joints. Also, out of guduchi, amritadi guggul is made, which works well for elevated uric acid levels.

4. Musta herb: This is another effective herb to control this condition. You can take coarse powder of musta, boiling it in water after soaking overnight. Filter it first before drinking.

5. Black raisins: Eating raisins is considered good for bone density and reduces the risk of arthritis and gout. You can soak 10 to 15 black raisins in water overnight and drink that water and chew the raisins the next morning.

If you can find an Ayurvedic physician in your local community or area, consult them for alternative therapies.

UNTREATED HYPERURICEMIA

Other than gout, the ramifications of hyperuricemia is quite diverse. We did touch upon hyperuricemia and its ramifications earlier in the book; now is the time to list these in more detail. Let's begin by asking the question "What damage or damages can asymptomatic and symptomatic hyperuricemia cause?" Here's a bird's eye view:

NONALCOHOLIC FATTY LIVER DISEASE

Since protein metabolism occurs in the liver and the end product uric acid is formed there, elevated levels of this uric acid left untreated have the potential to cause what is known as nonalcoholic fatty liver disease (NAFLD). NAFLD is defined as the accumulation of liver fat in people who drink little or no alcohol.

The cause of NAFLD is unknown. Risk factors include obesity, high cholesterol, and type 2 diabetes. Most people have no symptoms. In rare cases, people may experience fatigue or pain. Over time, inflammation and scarring of the liver (cirrhosis) can occur. The interesting point is that elevated serum uric acid levels (hyperuricemia—both symptomatic and asymptomatic) strongly reflect and may even cause oxidative stress in the liver for a person suffering from NAFLD.

Oxidative stress is a bodily condition that happens when antioxidant levels are low. These levels can be measured through blood plasma. When there is an imbalance between free radicals and antioxidant defenses, the body experiences oxidative stress. This oxidative stress triggers liver damage by altering lipids, proteins, and DNA (our genetic material) contents, but this is not all. NAFLD also causes insulin resistance. The hormone insulin helps control the amount of sugar in the blood. With insulin resistance, the body's cells don't respond normally to insulin. This stops glucose from entering the cells as easily, so it builds up in the blood. This can eventually lead to type 2 diabetes. In addition, dyslipidaemia (abnormal body fats) and metabolic syndrome are also considered risk factors for the progression of fatty liver disease.

METABOLIC SYNDROME

Metabolic syndrome, which we mentioned as a symptom of NAFLD, is also known as Syndrome X or MetS. A patient with metabolic syndrome shows multiple symptoms that may include sleep apnea, NAFLD, weight gain, heart disease, diabetes, and/or kidney disease. One feature that is common to patients with metabolic syndrome is an elevated uric acid level. Recent developments in science have evidence that elevated uric acid levels has direct correlation to MetS. This is because excess uric acid in the body has been correlated to excess body fat, thus leading to weight gain, obesity, and increased cholesterol levels.

This elevation also has a direct correlation with heart disease because, as discussed earlier, uric acid has the ability to cause systemic inflammation, which is inflammation that occurs when the immune system is constantly defending the body. Stress, infection, or chronic diseases can put the body in a pro-inflammatory state. When this happens, the immune system becomes primed and ready to create an inflammatory response. When caused by elevated uric acid levels, this response causes negative issues for the body, like coronary artery disease, which then leads to heart disease.

UNDERMINING THE EFFECTS OF NITROUS OXIDE

Elevated uric acid levels are also known to cause loss of vascular compliance and disruption of insulin-glucose correspondence. This is because elevated uric acid has been found to undermine the effects that nitrous oxide (NO) has on the body. NO is produced naturally by the body and has been found to cause vasodilation, which helps in circulation, thereby assisting in keeping blood pressure at normal levels.

In addition to this, NO has been found to help insulin move from the bloodstream to cells (specifically muscle cells), where glucose is converted to glycogen and stored. Undermining or bringing down levels of NO, therefore, leads to increased blood pressure or hypertension, as well as an increase in insulin resistance. It is interesting to note that fructose, purines, and alcohol cause elevation of uric acid, which then causes a reduction in levels of NO.

This undermining of the effects of NO also causes oxidative stress, damaging tissues and DNA, thus further inciting inflammation and leading to endothelial functional damage, which causes problems with the expression of the insulin gene and therefore has the potential to adversely affect its release in required quantities. Another adverse effect of reduced levels of NO in the body is erectile dysfunction in men, which is often treated by using drugs that cause an increase in nitrous oxide levels in the penile region.

THE URIC ACID HANDBOOK

HYPERTHYROIDISM

Patients suffering from thyroid dysfunction, specifically hyperthyroidism, have also been shown to suffer concurrently from gout. This leads us to believe that keeping uric acid to normal levels in patients suffering from issues of the thyroid is very important to ensure that they don't suffer from symptoms of a gout flare-up later.

AGING

A correlation has been found between hyperuricemia (asymptomatic or symptomatic) and aging. The enzyme called adenosine monophosphate-activated protein kinase (AMPK) is thought of as an antiaging enzyme. It is known to work as a cleanup agent for the cellular world that also maintains energy balance. Simply put, when AMPK is activated, it signals to the body that there is no need to store fat and compels it to hunt or scavenge. As a result, our hunter-gatherer ancestors became lean hunting predators. However, AMPK has a competitor that works against it. This enzyme is called Adenosine Monophosphate Deaminase 2 (AMPD2), which reduces fat burning and increases its storage. These two enzymes worked in complete unison, balancing each other during the hunter-gatherer days. We needed to feel less hungry and store fat, and at the same time, we needed to use fat to work and scavenge or hunt for food. Studies have found that when uric acid levels in the body go beyond normal levels, AMPD2 is activated. This activation of the AMPD2 leads to inhibition of AMPK and its positive effects, thus leading to an increase in the rate of aging.

GUT HEALTH

The gut maintains its health due to the presence of healthy and helpful gut bacteria. This gut bacteria needs lipopolysaccharide (LPS) to maintain its structure and health. Sometimes this LPS is known to get into the bloodstream due to a leaky gut and becomes an endotoxin (some sort of poison) for the body (i.e., it carries the toxins of the gut bacteria and releases them in the bloodstream). The important point to note here is that researchers have found that this gut leakage is often seen when elevated uric acid levels are observed in the blood. Not only this, but it has also been found that uric acid is secreted in the intestines as well, which promotes the decay of intestinal linings and, thus, a leaky gut. If left untreated, leaky gut often leads to immune disorders and negatively impacts skeletal muscles, the skin, the pancreas, the liver, and the brain. All the more reason to keep an eye on your uric acid levels.

DEMENTIA

A study conducted at Johns Hopkins School of Medicine found that uric acid levels in the high end of the normal range were more likely to be associated with cognitive problems, even when the researchers controlled for age, sex, weight, race, education, diabetes, hypertension, smoking, and alcohol abuse. These findings suggest that older people with serum (blood) uric acid levels in the high end of the normal range are more likely to process information slowly and experience failures of verbal and working memory, as measured by the Wechsler Adult Intelligence Scale and other well-established neuropsychological tests.[10]

"It might be useful for primary-care physicians to ask elderly adults with high-normal serum uric acid about any problems they might be having with their thinking, and perhaps refer those who express concern, or whose family members express concern, for neuropsychological screening," says lead author David Schretlen, PhD. "The link between high-normal uric acid and cognitive problems is also sufficiently intriguing for the authors to propose clinical studies of whether medicines that reduce uric acid, such as

---

10 David Schretlen, "High-Normal Uric Acid Linked with Mild Cognitive Impairment in the Elderly," American Psychological Association, last updated 2007, https://www.apa.org/news/press/releases/2007/01/uric-cognition#:~:text =High%2Dnormal%20uric%20acid%20levels,hypertension%2C%20smoking% 20and%20alcohol%20abuse.

allopurinol, can help older people with high-normal uric acid avoid developing the mild cognitive deficits that often precede dementia. For reasons that are not entirely clear, uric acid levels increase with age," says Dr. Schretlen.[11]

He also says there is mounting evidence that end-stage renal (kidney) disease increases the risk of cognitive dysfunction and dementia in elderly adults. Given this web of connections, uric acid could potentially become a valuable biological marker for very early cognitive problems in old age. The researchers say that it's unclear why mild cognitive problems appear with high-normal uric acid because, paradoxically, it also has antioxidant properties that are thought to be protective in other situations.

CANCERS

In recent years, metabolic syndrome has been a hot topic among medical scientists. As discussed earlier, MetS indicates a cluster of metabolic abnormalities, including abdominal fat, insulin resistance, hyperglycemia, hypertension, and dyslipidemia. Increasing evidence has shown that MetS has a close relationship with the incidence and development of some specific cancers, such as breast cancer, ovarian cancer, and pancreatic cancer. We have already mentioned how as a contributory factor of MetS, hyperuricemia plays an essential role in the formation of various metabolic disorders, including diabetes, obesity, hypertension, and so on.

While it is assumed that MetS and cancer share common underlying mechanisms of oxidative stress and inflammation, evidence is now emerging that hyperuricemia can be another potent detrimental factor, too.

When Uric acid is present at its normal levels, its scavenging of free radicals reduces the risk of cancer. On the other hand, uric acid in very high concentrations may trigger inflammatory stress, and it may

---

11 David Schretlen, "High-Normal Uric Acid."

also have intracellular pro-oxidative activity. Pro-oxidative activity is the opposite of the scavenging activity (immunity stimulation) that uric acid displays when present at normal levels in the blood. A pro-oxidant environment confers a growth advantage to tumor cells and influences carcinogenic potential by stimulating specific processes that regulate cell growth.

Increasing numbers of studies have recently suggested that a high uric acid level is associated with higher cancer incidence and mortality. In fact, a statistically significant association has been found between higher uric acid levels and increased mortality of total cancers, especially the specific sites of digestive cancer, which is also more significant in females than males. For colorectal cancer (CRC), it was found that uric acid levels gradually increased from stage I to stage IV, suggesting that the uric acid level reflected the severity of CRC. In addition, an elevated serum level of uric acid was shown to be a significant marker for an additional malignant growth in lymph nodes in patients with colon cancer.

Among pancreatic cancer patients, it was also observed that elevated uric acid levels were an independent poor prognostic factor for overall survival. In addition to its association with the development of digestive cancer, uric acid levels also correlate with the incidence of urological cancers. It was found that gout patients had a higher risk of prostate cancer, followed by bladder and renal cancers.[12]

It is also not rare for cancer patients, especially patients with leukemia, to have high uric acid level. As for respiratory organs, it has been found that among lung cancer patients with higher uric acid levels, there was a higher percentage of cancers that then showed up in the brain, which obviously led to lower overall survival.

---

12 Shuyi Mi, Liang Gong, and Ziqi Sui, "Friend or Foe? An Unrecognized Role of Uric Acid in Cancer Development and the Potential Anticancer Effects of Uric Acid-lowering Drugs," *Journal of Cancer* 11, no. 17 (2020): 5236–5244, doi: 10.7150/jca.46200.

Gout, which is characterized by symptomatic hyperuricemia, is also considered a risk factor for cancer. Additional evidence has shown that gout increases the risk of cancer, and a higher incidence of all causes of cancer has been found in the high prevalence of various gout-related comorbidities. A nationwide population study investigating the relationship between gout and cancer found that the annual incidence of cancer in gout patients was more than double that of the average population.[13]

We now know the potential role of uric acid in cancer initiation and progression, and it makes for good reading to know that now, uric acid–lowering drugs have the potential for treating such cancers. This can be explained by the fact that in cancer chemotherapy, drugs that disrupt microtubule dynamics are used widely by clinicians. Microtubules are narrow, hollow tube-like structures found in the cytoplasm (the fluid inside a cell) of plant and animal cells. Their main function is to help support the shape of a cell and help genetic material move easily between cells. These microtubules play an essential role in keeping our cells healthy.

Scientists have recently deduced that microtubules could now be considered an ideal target for anticancer drugs because of their essential role in mitosis, the process in which one cell divides into two genetically identical daughter cells. To simplify things, just consider this: It is an ironic fact that the same microtubules that maintain cell structures can sometimes also induce uncontrolled cell duplication that encourages cancerous growth.

A drug by the name colchicine used to treat acute gout attacks by reducing the inflammation caused by crystals of uric acid in the joints also possesses microtubule-disruption activities, thus providing anticancer effects to the therapy. It is now understood that colchicine can inhibit the cell duplication properties of microtubules,

---

13 Wang et al., "Increased Risk of Cancer in Relation to Gout," *Mediators of Inflammation* (2015): 680853, https://pubmed.ncbi.nlm.nih.gov/26504360.

which leads to prolonged arrest in the growth of cancer cells. Thus, its anticancer role as a microtubule inhibitor has made colchicine a drug of choice in many anticancer treatments. In some studies, researchers have used colchicine as an anticancer drug to inhibit colon and liver cancer cells.

Other commonly used uric acid-lowering agents are the previously mentioned allopurinol and febuxostat. These drugs are considered very effective in bringing down levels of uric acid in the body and reducing oxidative stress caused by elevated uric acid levels. It is basically the property of the two drugs of bringing down UA levels that gives them their anticancer activity. It is encouraging, therefore, to know that researchers have now shown that long-term (> 1 year) use of allopurinol has resulted in a 34 to 36 percent decrease in the risk of developing prostate cancer.

We have mentioned that elevated uric acid levels cause NAFLD. Treating NAFLD by bringing down uric acid levels may effectively help allopurinol to provide protection against growth of cancer cells in the liver. In addition to lowering blood glucose levels, oxidative stress, and inflammation in the liver, allopurinol can inhibit fat deposition on the cancer cells and thus any probability of cancer growth. As for febuxostat, in addition to its ability to lower levels of serum uric acid, it also has a high ability to reduce oxidative stress, thus indicating that it may have strong anticancer potential.

In conclusion, inflammation induced by elevated UA and urate crystals, as well as oxidative stress during the interaction between uric acid and the immune system, is thought to constitute the underlying mechanism stimulating the growth of cancer cells. In the presence of high UA levels, the spread of cancer to other organs from the liver (which is a frequent site where cancers first happen because of its unique biological characteristics) is always a very high possibility. To some extent, hyperuricemia may promote this by affecting the liver microenvironment by causing NAFLD.

Sustained exposure to inflammatory stimuli and oxidation induced by elevated uric acid may also lead to the formation of local immunosuppression in the liver, providing a relatively tolerant liver microenvironment that allows the survival and growth of foreign tumor cells. By inducing oxidative stress in both liver and pancreatic cells, hyperuricemia can result in the development of insulin resistance and growth inhibition, which is associated with increased fat deposition in the liver, which then may lead to the development of malignant tumors.

Alternatively, elevated uric acid can also originate from fructose metabolism, and when fructose is metabolized, there is a transient decrease in ATP (energy) levels, which induces oxidative stress and cellular dysfunction, thus playing a pivotal role in increased fat deposition in the liver, which leads to malfunction in the overall metabolic processes happening there. Because this is linked with liver cell injury and inflammation, liver cells may get inflamed, causing NAFLD, which, if left untreated, becomes a fertile microenvironment for the growth and multiplication of cancer cells.

Now here is the clincher. We need to be careful in concluding that hyperuricemia causes cancer. This is because the role of hyperuricemia as an independent risk factor for the initiation and progression of cancer is still considered controversial, and its effect may markedly differ according to sex. Scientists and researchers are suggesting that an increased uric acid level might be a valuable marker (a marker found in blood, urine, or body tissues that can be elevated by the presence of one or more types of cancer) rather than an independent risk factor or even a carcinogenic substance itself. However, we should also accept that an increase in UA levels beyond what is considered normal indicates a lifestyle at increased risk for cancer. Having said that, it is essential to note that some clinicians associate gout and symptoms of breast cancer, while others say that there is a higher risk for male gout patients developing prostate cancer. Studies are on to ascertain a precise determination of the relationship between high UA and cancer development, particularly in relation to sex and specific sites of malignancies.

Hyperuricemia may also contribute to the metastasis of some cancers, but the precise mechanism of this happening is still being studied by research teams worldwide. This may lead to the development of many medicines in the future. Your clinician may not know the extent to which they should try to lower uric acid, though many researchers suggest that UA levels of up to 7mg/dL in males and 6mg/dL in females are considered safe with respect to mortality. We can, therefore, safely say that existing drugs like allopurinol and febuxostat used to bring down levels of uric acid may be a novel strategy for the management of some refractory (cancer that does not respond to treatment) cancers, but the application of those drugs is still being evaluated at this juncture.[14]

14 Shuyi Mi, *Journal of Cancer*, 5236–5244.

THE URIC ACID HANDBOOK

CHAPTER 3

LIFESTYLE VS. LIFE STAGE

Are you eating a diet rich in red meat and shellfish and drinking beverages sweetened with fructose? Is your alcohol consumption, especially of beer, regular? Your lifestyle may be inviting hyper-uricemia into your life. Making a lifestyle change is challenging, especially when you want to transform many things simultaneously. We suggest changing your perspective on how you view this change. Let's try to imagine that it's an evolution.

Lifestyle changes take time and require support from various sources. When ready to make the change, we understand that the difficult part is committing and following through. We suggest that you do your research and make a plan to prepare you for success. Planning means setting small goals and taking things one step at a time.

Here are some tips to help you make lasting, positive lifestyle and behavioral changes.

Your plan is a map that will guide you on this journey of change. Think of it as an adventure. When making the plan, be specific. Detail the time of day you can take walks and how long you'll walk. How will you change your week's menu? Now, write everything down, and ask yourself if you're confident that these activities and goals are realistic for you.

Start small. After you've identified realistic short-term and long-term goals, break down your goals into small, manageable steps that are specifically defined and can be measured. Is your long-term goal to lose 20 pounds within the next five months? In this case, an excellent weekly goal would be to lose 1 pound a week. If you would like to eat healthier, consider as a goal for the week replacing dessert with a healthier option, like fruit or yogurt. At the end of the week, you'll feel successful knowing you met your goal.

Change one behavior at a time. Unhealthy behaviors develop over the course of time, so replacing them with healthy ones requires time, too. We run into problems when we try to change too much too fast. To succeed, focus on one goal or change at a time. As new healthy behaviors become a habit, try to add another goal that works toward the overall change.

Do you have a buddy? A friend, coworker, or family member, or someone else on your journey will keep you motivated and focused. Perhaps it can be someone who will go to the gym with you or someone who is also trying to quit alcohol. Talk about what you are doing and what you would like to do. A support group may be a good idea. Having someone with whom to share your struggles and successes makes the work easier and the mission less intimidating.

Accept help! Those who care about you and will listen strengthen your resilience and commitment. If you feel overwhelmed or unable to meet your goals by yourself, consider seeking help. Psychologists are uniquely trained to understand the connection between the mind and body, as well as the factors that promote behavioral change. Asking for help doesn't necessarily mean a lifetime of therapy; even just a few sessions can help you examine and set attainable goals or address the emotional issues that may be getting in your way.

WHAT IS THE CHANGE THAT YOU NEED TO COMMIT TO?

Large-scale studies have clarified several long-suspected relations between lifestyle factors, hyperuricemia, and gout, including purine-rich foods, dairy foods, various beverages, fructose, and vitamin C supplementation. Furthermore, recent studies have identified the substantial burden of comorbidities among patients with hyperuricemia and gout.

BEVERAGES

How often do you indulge in alcohol? If the answer is, "Often," then read on. The association between alcohol and hyperuricemia is well known. The type and amount both affect the serum uric acid level. A recent study showed that the prevalence of hyperuricemia increases proportionally with alcohol consumption in male drinkers, with an approximately 1.7-fold higher risk of hyperuricemia in heavy drinkers than nondrinkers.[15] Interestingly, prevalence rates did not differ much among drinkers and nondrinkers in the female population. The study revealed that uric acid levels increased with beer or liquor intake but not with wine, with maximal increase noted with beer consumption. Beer has something called guanosine that contributes to this increase in uric acid levels.

FRUCTOSE

What is the connection between the sugars added to approximately 74 percent of the foods and beverages sold in America's grocery

---

15 Zhao Li et al., "The Relation of Moderate Alcohol Consumption to Hyperuricemia in a Rural General Population," *International Journal of Environmental Research and Public Health* 13, no. 7 (2016): 732; Hyon K. Choi and Gary Curhan, "Beer, Liquor, and Wine Consumption and Serum Uric Acid Level: The Third National Health and Nutrition Examination Survey," *Arthritis and Rheumatism* 51, no. 6 (2004): 1023–1029, DOI: 10.1002/art.20821.

stores and the ever-increasing rates of chronic degenerative diseases, including the impact on mental faculties?[16]

We mentioned that our ancestors lived and subsisted on a diet that consisted mainly of fruits. As they ate fruits, their bodies converted that into fructose, which then converted to fats and ensured that energy was stored in that form to be burned during times of need and various activities. The fructose thus formed after ingesting fruits didn't cause overeating and, therefore, didn't elevate uric acid levels.

In addition, many fruits contain nutrients like potassium, flavanols, fiber, and vitamin C, which can offset or counter any potential rise in uric acid levels. This is true even today. Modern humans still get fructose from fruits, honey, and some vegetables like broccoli, asparagus, okra, and artichokes. However, we have complicated matters a bit. First, we have begun to use table sugar quite frequently. Our consumption has fallen by about 30 percent when compared with what we consumed in the 1970s, and most consumers today know that added sugar is toxic, taking steps to reduce added sugar by not adding extra sugar to their coffee or by opting for foods with labels that say "no added sugar." Still, at 60 pounds per person per year, our consumption is very high compared to that of our ancestors, who never had sugar in their few million years of existence. Very recently (about a thousand years ago), we began to manufacture sugar from sugarcane and beetroot.

Table sugar is chemically classified as a disaccharide—two molecules of simple sugars that come together to form the disaccharide sucrose. This further breaks down into fructose and glucose (both monosaccharides) in the small intestine, aided in large measure by the enzyme sucrase (do you still remember uricase, the enzyme that helped break down uric acid into allantoic acid and ammonia that's

---

16 "Hidden in Plain Sight," SugarScience.edu, accessed October 12, 2022, https://sugarscience.ucsf.edu/hidden-in-plain-sight.

very easily excreted by the kidneys? Well just like uricase in the case of uric acid, sucrose needs sucrase to break down).

While glucose's primary role is to break down and produce energy, fructose, as we now know, stores itself as body fat until it is burned by the body for energy. This leaves us with more fructose than we can possibly digest because the fructose from table sugar now becomes an extra, as we are still getting fructose from fruits, honey and vegetables like our ancestors did in the ancient world. As we ingest more fructose, we also increase our fat stores. Add to this our sedentary lifestyles, which also adds to the burden. This is due to the fact that our energy requirements have shrunk by quite a large amount today, as the need to forage, scavenge, or hunt for food are no longer necessary for our subsistence. These are now replaced by the time we spent looking at our smartphones or working on laptops or watching Netflix on TV screens.

Now that we've discussed the role that table sugar plays in the high rates of obesity and weight gain in our society, let's look at another problem: the quantity of fructose we are ingesting in the form of high fructose corn syrup (HFCS). Think soft drinks, processed and junk foods, and pastries and desserts. This includes the sauces or ketchups that we add to our burgers, chicken sandwiches, and pizza; and snack foods like cookies, candies, crackers, jellies, jams, cereals, and sweetened yogurt. Close your eyes and think of all these and much more, then visualize that each of them contain HFCS, which further unbalances the effect of ghrelin and leptin to fuel even more hunger as the influence of ghrelin rises to more than required levels. This makes us eat more such food that contains HFCS, so much so that unknown to us, per capita consumption of high fructose corn syrup in the United States is 36.7 pounds.[17]

---

17 "Per Capita Consumption of High Fructose Corn Syrup in the United States from 2000 to 2019," Statista, last accessed November 28, 2022, https://www.statista.com/statistics/328893/per-capita-consumption-of-high-fructose-corn-syrup-in-the-us.

HFCS works like a cloaked killer. On one end it makes us follow the hedonistic pathway by asking us to eat when we don't really need to, and on the other it disarms the starvation pathway by encouraging mindless eating. This results in a vicious cycle of excessive eating, leading to weight gain, hypertension, insulin resistance, and elevated blood sugar, and the body holding onto fat in the false belief that it is starving. So our fat stores increase and the body has to contend with a resultant rise in uric acid levels. The relationship between fructose metabolism, or breakdown, and elevated levels of uric acid is well established.

This hidden assassin stealthily attacks us from many angles. Keep in mind that the fructose in HFCS is primarily metabolized in the liver and the kidneys. Like uric acid and sucrose, fructose needs the enzyme fructokinase to further break down into fat stores. As fructokinase helps in the breakdown of fructose in the liver and kidneys, it also depletes ATP by 40 to 50 percent. This depletion is very bad news for other processes in the body. It leads to the inhibition of protein synthesis, which can cause oxidative stress and over time lead to the development of cardiovascular disease. It also causes an overall dysfunction in the mitochondria (the place in our cells where production of energy occurs) and, as a result, our cells scream to us that they are running out of energy. Our body therefore gets into an energy-preservation mode. As metabolism slows, less fat is burned from our fat stores and more incoming calories are produced by more food ingestion, which in turn leads to more than the required amount of fat storage. Not only this, fructose is also known to stimulate triglyceride synthesis, increasing fat deposits in the liver and the risk factors for developing cardiovascular disease.

So what's all this got to do with elevated uric acid levels? Well the bad news is that fructose stimulates the production of uric acid as it goes about depleting the amount of ATP energy molecules. The enzyme fructokinase, released to help in fructose metabolism, also pushes the body to create more uric acid. This causes oxidative stress in the pancreas, specifically on those cells that produce insulin, thus causing an increase in insulin resistance. It also leads to a reduction in nitric oxide (NO) synthesis, which is so very important for our vascular health. As a result we become more prone to developing lifestyle disorders like hypertension, cardiovascular disease, and erectile dysfunction.

WHAT'S YOUR SUGAR QUOTIENT?

Sugar-sweetened beverage consumption is associated with increased serum uric acid level, and an increase in mean urate level by 0.42 mg/dL was observed in those who consumed four or more servings of sugar-sweetened beverages per day.[18] Fructose, specifically as part of the high-fructose corn syrup used as an industrial sweetener in these sugar-sweetened beverages, emerged as a major contributory factor toward hyperuricemia over past two decades.

Excess fructose in the system also leads to high cognitive impairment as we age, which might develop into Alzheimer's disease and/or dementia down the road. This impairment is also due to less synthesis of NO in the brain, which leads to impairment of memory function and of transmission of messages within the brain.

In conclusion, we can, therefore, safely say that fructose-induced hyperuricemia has direct and indirect effects on many of us developing metabolic syndrome or MetS.

---

18 Ramesh Aggarwal et al., "Hyperuricemia: A Lifestyle Change," *Urology and Nephrology Open Access Journal* 6, no. 6 (2018), https://medcraveonline.com/UNOAJ/hyperuricemia-a-lifestyle-change.html.

Lead intoxication also leads to hyperuricemia and gout. This association was highlighted in the era of prohibition in the US, when "moonshine," or illegal homemade liquor, was brewed in lead-lined vessels. This effect has also been noted today in populations living in areas with high levels of lead pollution.

Keeping all the currently available knowledge in mind, recommendations for lifestyle modification in hyper-uricemia are to avoid organ meats, high-fructose corn syrup in food and beverages, and alcohol overuse (defined as more than two servings per day for males and more than one serving per day for females.) Consume a limited intake of red meat and seafood intake, naturally sweetened fruit juice, table sugar, salt, and alcohol. We highly recommend increased intake of low-fat or nonfat dairy products and vegetables.

When it comes to HFCS-laced foods, researchers have found that kids with ADHD have elevated uric acid levels. They have deduced that this is also due to the HFCSs negatively impairing the dopamine receptors in the brain. These dopamine receptors release dopamine, which is another hormone classified as a type of neurotransmitter. Our body makes it, and our nervous system and brain use it to send messages between nerve cells. Dopamine is known as the "feel-good" hormone. It gives us a sense of pleasure and the motivation to do something when we are feeling pleasure. Dopamine is part of our reward system, and when this is impaired, kids show signs of ADHD.

The time to limit the use of table sugar laced with sucrose and strip HFCS from our lives is now!

MEAT AND SEAFOOD

It was found that serum uric acid increased by a mean of 0.48 mg/dL in the highest quintile of meat intake, and by 0.16 mg/dL in the highest quintile of seafood intake.[19] Total protein intake was not independently related to hyperuricemia, and surprisingly neither was purine-rich vegetable intake (peas, mushroom, lentils, spinach); all of these dietary practices were traditionally believed to be contributory. Low-fat dairy, specifically milk and yogurt, were found to be negatively associated with uric acid levels, with a difference approaching -0.21mg/dL for total dairy intake.

HYPERURICEMIA IN CHILDREN

Recently, the prevalence of hyperuricemia has markedly increased among children worldwide. Many clinical and epidemiological studies have suggested that increased serum uric acid levels may be closely associated with metabolic syndrome, chronic kidney disease, and cardiovascular disease. Obesity is another major cause of hyperuricemia in otherwise healthy children and adolescents. Obesity is often accompanied by metabolic syndrome; hyperuricemia in obese children and adolescents is associated with the components of metabolic syndrome and noncommunicable diseases, including hypertension, insulin resistance, dyslipidaemia, and chronic kidney disease. Treatment strategies for hyperuricemia include lifestyle intervention and drug administration.

Hyperuricemia in children has become a significant public health issue and is currently gaining more and more attention. Chronic kidney disease causes a substantial burden to individuals, families, and health-care systems due to the reduced quality of life and the need for dialysis and even kidney transplantation. Hyperuricemia

---

19 Hyon K. Choi, *Arthritis and Rheumatism*, 1023–1029.

and chronic kidney disease probably influence one another in many ways, depending on multiple mechanisms. However, what factors may be associated with hyperuricemia and chronic kidney disease in children remain uncertain.

It is vital to understand that the measurement of the serum uric acid level, most commonly considered in adult patients, is frequently obtained inadvertently for pediatric patients. Most standard references for average uric acid values do not consider the impact of the metabolic changes in children at different ages on the uric acid level. A substantial number of childhood conditions may produce alarming results in the serum uric acid level. Knowledge of normal serum uric acid levels and of the conditions affecting those levels in children enables a more focused pursuit of underlying abnormalities.

The reference ranges for uric acid in the blood are as follows:[20]

Child: 2.5 to 5.5 mg/dL or 0.12 to 0.32 mmol/L

Newborn: 2.0 to 6.2 mg/dL

Various factors are responsible for hyperuricemia in children; however, minimal data is available. Patients with preexisting conditions like congenital heart disease, asthma, epilepsy, nephrotic syndrome, and cancers should routinely be screened for hyperuricemia and managed accordingly to avoid long-term complications.

Some acute or chronic conditions that can be a significant causative factor of increased uric acid in children and adolescents are Down syndrome, congenital heart diseases, metabolic or genetic diseases, gastroenteritis, bronchial asthma, and malignant disorders. Obesity is one of the significant causes of hyperuricemia because of its association with metabolic disorders and non-communicable diseases like hypertension, insulin resistance, dyslipidaemia, and

---

20 Kathleen Deska Pagana, Timothy J. Pagana, and Theresa N. Pagana, *Mosby's Diagnostic & Laboratory Test Reference*, 14th ed., St. Louis, MO: Elsevier, 2019.

THE URIC ACID HANDBOOK

chronic kidney disease.[21] Literature has reported high prevalence of elevated uric acid levels in the obese population than the general population and proved a direct association of increased BMI with elevated uric acid. Another study in China has shown a high prevalence of hyperuricemia in children ages three to six years, of the male gender, and a strong association with high diastolic blood pressure and increased triglycerides concentration.

Hyperuricemia can also occur as a side effect of several drugs like some antiepileptics, with valproate and phenobarbital being the commonest ones; thiazide diuretics, cyclosporine, theophylline, and pyrazinamide have also been reported as the main causative factors, with their mechanism not fully understood.[22]

WALKING AND EXERCISE AFTER A GOUT FLARE-UP

While exercising is important, it is crucial to understand and love your body. Multiple joints in your body may be affected if you have suffered a recent gout flare-up. Quickly diving into a rigorous exercise regimen may be more harmful than expected. Go slow and choose the right type of exercise.

---

21 Masaru Kubota, "Hyperuricemia in Children and Adolescents: Present Knowledge and Future Directions," *Journal of Nutrition and Metabolism* (2019): 3480718, doi: 10.1155/2019/3480718; Erika Kuwahara et al., "Increased Childhood BMI Is Associated with Young Adult Serum Uric Acid Levels: A Linkage Study From Japan," *Pediatric Research* 81, no. 2 (2017): 293–298, doi: 10.1038/pr.2016.213; Nan Li et al., "Prevalence of Hyperuricemia and Its Related Risk Factors among Preschool Children from China," *Science Reports* 7, no. 1 (2017): 9448, doi: 10.1038/s41598-017-10120-8.

22 Johannes Trück et al., "Gout in Pediatric Renal Transplant Recipients," *Pediatric Nephrology* 25 (2010): 2535–2538, doi.org/10.1007/s00467-010 -1599-6.

After a gout flare-up subsides, waterborne exercises may be an excellent way to start reengaging in exercise because the buoyancy of the water will reduce the impact on the joints.

You should be careful not to overdo it once you ease into post-flare exercise. Look out for symptoms like pain coming back in your joints when walking once the flare-up has subsided. If you experience such pain with walking after a flare-up, it is advisable to go back to using walking support and reducing your planned exercise until the pain subsides. Listen to the cues your body gives you.

EXPERT TIPS FOR EXERCISING WITH GOUT

Having gout doesn't mean you can't be active or even run regularly. The key is to increase your workout intensity gradually. Consult your physician and physical therapist before starting any exercise routine. Here are five gout-friendly workout tips to start moving, and keep moving, with gout:

1. Choose the right footwear: Because gout often affects the big toe, mid-foot, and ankle, choosing suitable footwear is essential. A physical therapist can help evaluate the best footwear for gout patients. It has been observed that specialized footwear benefits patients by changing the leg and foot's alignment, influencing the foot muscles' activity, and influencing your gait pattern. These modifications work toward decreasing the pressure on our joints.

2. Follow a comfortable walking pace: Remember, your goal is to move without pain. So listen to your body. You must start slowly, using a walking pace that creates the least stress and pressure. As you begin to feel comfortable with your walking stride, you could test a faster pace that increases your heart rate.

THE URIC ACID HANDBOOK

3. Include other low-impact aerobic exercises: Beyond walking, it is good to consider adding different heart-pumping activities into your regular aerobic exercise, such as swimming or riding a stationary bike. Both are excellent options for gout patients because they don't put as much pressure on the weight-bearing joints of the feet, ankles, and knees. Likewise, an elliptical machine can be a wise choice to get your arms and legs moving without excessive joint force.

4. Stretch your affected joint: Once your gout flare-up subsides, you may want to regain flexibility in the joint to ensure ease of movement. Most physical therapists recommend simple stretching by moving your joints forward, backward, and around to a comfortable limit. Try to begin with a repetition of five and then gradually increase these repetitions.

5. Build muscle with strength exercises: Strong muscles can protect joints from wear and tear, especially for joints affected by gout. Beyond weight training, simple resistance exercises (exercises that use your body weight) can effectively build muscle. For example, try an elastic resistance band by holding each end and putting your foot in the middle, then repeating your flexibility exercises while pushing against the force of the band.

The key with any exercise after a gout flare-up is to go slow and listen to your body.

STRESS MANAGEMENT

How are your stress levels? For some people, stress can trigger gout attacks. That's because high levels of stress and anxiety are associated with increased uric acid levels. Taking action to manage your stress can also support a calmer state of mind and reduce the inflammation associated with stress. When you are stressed out, your body loses pantothenic acid. This acid is vital because it aids the body in removing uric acid, and when levels of pantothenic acid are low, uric acid is high, which leads to gout.

It's hard to avoid stress, whether caused by work, relationships, or any other factor, but when that stress is long-term, it can be a trigger for elevated levels of uric acid.

Diaphragmatic breathing is a technique that involves a steady inhale while expanding the belly and a long exhale while bringing the belly in. This technique can help you relieve stress in a moment.

Gauge your stress levels by using the Stress Indicators Questionnaire on page 65.

Yoga and meditation also reduce stress and make it easier to manage daily challenges.

YOGA

Doing low-impact exercises while going through a gout flare-up or increased uric acid levels can be beneficial. Once the intensity of that flare-up reduces, these exercises could provide you with relief by decreasing pain and improving mobility.

Yoga reduces stress, fosters mental calmness, and teaches coping techniques, such as breathing exercises, which may help you manage pain and depression. Clinicians and physical therapists believe that patients who suffer from elevated levels of uric acid or gout and do yoga daily under supervision show significant improvement in pain levels, flexibility, and psychological health.

HOW TO BEGIN DOING YOGA

It would be best if you first met with your health-care provider to ensure that yoga is compatible with your condition. Generally speaking, most physical therapists will advise any beginner against trying to start a yoga practice on their own.

A gentle class for beginners is an excellent place to start. Calling a yoga studio in your city, describing the problem and challenges, and then asking for teacher information is a good place to begin. There are so many different yoga styles and teacher-training programs that yoga teachers' expertise varies greatly. Therefore, you need to find a knowledgeable teacher to offer you modifications when necessary.

An out-of-the-box approach could be trying to find a prenatal yoga class since this is gentle, will be sensitive to joint problems, and offers individualized attention. If you plan to try a class for seniors or a prenatal class but are neither elderly nor pregnant, be sure to contact the teacher ahead of time to ensure they feel comfortable having you in class. Most teachers will be amenable when you explain your reasons for wanting to attend. Though you will need to be more selective in your choice of classes, there is information about basic poses, equipment, and etiquette that will help you feel more comfortable as you begin.

WHAT KIND OF YOGA?

If, for some reason, you cannot find a teacher with the specific experience you seek, you needn't despair. Here are some styles of yoga that emphasize rehabilitation and adaptation. If you research each of them and stay watchful while practicing them, the physical limitations you experience due to gout can begin to be circumvented. But the advice remains to keep your health-care provider informed.

In any case, the key is to go slowly and keep listening to your body as you perform the yogic poses, and to stop any posture or movement immediately if that causes pain. Here is a list of some yoga methods that could be researched and selected through trial under expert supervision.

- Chair yoga makes yoga accessible to people who cannot stand for long periods or come down to the mat.
- Water yoga is excellent for people with joint pain.

- Viniyoga is intended to be adaptive, tailoring a practice that is appropriate to each individual's physical condition, even within a group practice setting.
- Iyengar yoga pioneered props to support the body in finding comfort in poses while maintaining good alignment. Iyengar teachers are very well trained in anatomy and pose modification.
- Anusara is an option for people with more mobility who want to do a more active practice. Taking inspiration from Iyengar's methods, Anusara teachers are highly trained in alignment and adaptation.
- Kripalu and Sivananda are gentle practices that are appropriate for beginners and allow one to do things at one's own pace.

The following yoga asanas, or poses, when practiced regularly, can not only help reduce uric acid but prevent uric acid crystals from depositing in the joints, remove them, and help prevent a flare-up.

- Ardha Matsyendrasana (Half Spinal Twist Pose)
- Bhujangasana (Cobra Pose)
- Dhanurasana (Bow Pose)
- Halasana (Plow Pose)
- Hastashirasana (Hand-to-Head Pose)
- Januhastasana (Hand-to-Knee Pose)
- Makarasana (Crocodile Pose)
- Pavanamukhtasana (Wind-Relieving Pose)
- Pranayama (Breathing technique)
- Tadasana (Mountain Pose)
- Trikonasana (Triangle Pose)
- Uttana Padasana (Extended Leg Pose)
- Veerasana (Hero Pose)
- Vrikshasana (Tree Pose)

So, awaken the yogi in you, practice these asanas every day, and lead a healthy life by keeping your uric acid levels within the normal range.

GETTING A MASSAGE FOR GOUT RELIEF

Is a massage suitable for gout? It can be!

As gout is inflammatory, an anti-inflammatory relief massage may be beneficial. Different massage techniques, such as Thai massage and those aimed at helping flush toxins from your body, are most helpful when getting a massage for gout.

If going to a massage therapist while suffering from gout symptoms doesn't sound like an ideal situation, you could consider the benefits of owning a massage chair, instead. You can also opt for massage therapy at home, getting a massage for gout in private and whenever you experience an attack. Massage chairs with foot and leg massage features are ideal. Massage chairs that provide additional services such as heat therapy and zero gravity reclining capabilities may also help treat gout effectively.

Some of the ways getting a massage for gout can help include:

1. Increasing blood circulation to reduce inflammation

2. Pain relief

3. Stress management

INCREASING BLOOD CIRCULATION

Massage has been shown to help increase blood flow. This betters blood circulation, helps alleviate inflammation, and improves joint health. As gout attacks the joints in our body (most commonly in the foot, ankle, or knee), this benefit of massage therapy tops the list!

As blood flows more efficiently through the body, it lessens inflammation around joints while delivering oxygen and nutrients to heal tissue that may be damaged. Increased circulation is the source of many benefits of massage therapy. If you are unable to get to a massage therapist, then you can look for lymphatic drainage self-massage. This type of massage technique is one of the best for increasing blood flow and the movement of lymph within the body, which helps flush toxins. Lymphatic drainage self-massage does take time to learn and should be done under expert supervision.

PAIN RELIEF

The pain relief experienced by getting a massage may also benefit gout symptoms since one of the primary aims of getting a massage for gout in the first place is pain relief.

STRESS MANAGEMENT

Stress management is a top method for treating gout symptoms naturally. Stress can trigger a gout attack or exacerbate symptoms if one is already in the midst of an attack. Unfortunately, this forms a sort of bilateral negative impact as pain from a gout attack can cause additional stress, enhancing the pain from the gout attack.

There are some easy ways to manage stress. For example, a massage for gout symptoms can offer deep relaxation and pain relief, which helps alleviate stress. Researchers have shown that even five minutes of hand or foot massaging profoundly affect a patient's perceived stress and anxiety levels. Other techniques that can be used during a massage include meditation or listening to calming music. Meditation during massage may help increase its effects on stress management. Mindfulness meditation is one of the most common forms of meditation practiced in tandem with getting a massage for anxiety and stress.

Getting massage for gout may help you treat symptoms and get back to remission as quickly as possible. However, professional advice is essential. If you are experiencing a gout attack and considering massage, you should first consult a doctor to see if it may be beneficial and safe.

STRESS INDICATORS QUESTIONNAIRE

This questionnaire will show how stress affects different parts of your life. Circle the response that best indicates how often you experience each stress indicator during a typical week.

When you have answered all the questions add the point totals for each section.

5: Almost always (five days a week)

4: Most of the time (three days a week)

3: Some of the time (one and one-half days a week)

2: Almost never (less than two hours a week)

1: Never

PERSONAL PROFILE

Gender: ❏ Male
       ❏ Female
      ❏ _____

Age: _____

Educational qualification: _____

Marital status: ❏ Married
        ❏ Unmarried

Salary: _____

Experience: _____

Present position: _____

The above data is going to be handy when you meet your doctor or counselor for a discussion about your stress levels. Additionally, this questionnaire, when filled out from time to time, can show changes in your life over time that may be causing you stress, such as changes in marital status, job status, or positions.

PHYSICAL INDICATORS

Particulars
1. My body feels tense all over.
2. I have a nervous sweat or sweaty palms.
3. I have a hard time feeling really relaxed.
4. I have severe or chronic lower back pain.
5. I get severe or chronic headaches.
6. I get tension or muscle spasms in my face, jaw, neck, or shoulders.
7. My stomach quivers or feels upset.
8. I get skin rashes or itching.
9. I have problems with my bowels (constipation, diarrhea).
10. I need to urinate more than most people.
11. My ulcer bothers me.
12. I feel short of breath after mild exercise like climbing up four flights of stairs.
13. Compared to most people, I have a very small or a very large appetite.
14. My weight is more than 15 pounds above what is recommended for a person my height and build.
15. I smoke tobacco.
16. I get sharp chest pains when I'm physically active.
17. I lack physical energy.
18. When I'm resting, my heart beats more than 100 times a minute.
19. Because of my busy schedule, I miss at least two meals during the week.
20. I don't really plan my meals for balanced nutrition.
21. I spend less than three hours a week getting vigorous physical exercise (running, playing basketball, tennis, swimming, etc.).

THE URIC ACID HANDBOOK

Almost Always	Most of the Time	Some of the Time	Almost Never	Never
5	4	3	2	1
5	4	3	2	1
5	4	3	2	1
5	4	3	2	1
5	4	3	2	1
5	4	3	2	1
5	4	3	2	1
5	4	3	2	1
5	4	3	2	1
5	4	3	2	1
5	4	3	2	1
5	4	3	2	1
5	4	3	2	1
5	4	3	2	1
5	4	3	2	1
5	4	3	2	1
5	4	3	2	1
5	4	3	2	1
5	4	3	2	1
5	4	3	2	1
5	4	3	2	1

Physical indicators point total: _____

BEHAVIORAL INDICATORS

Particulars
1. I stutter or get tongue-tied when I talk to other people.
2. I try to work while I'm eating lunch.
3. I have to work late.
4. I go to work even when I feel sick.
5. I have to bring work home.
6. I drink alcohol or use drugs to relax.
7. I have more than two beers, eight ounces of wine, or three ounces of hard liquor a day.
8. When I drink, I like to get really drunk.
9. I get drunk or "high" with other drugs more than once a week.
10. When I'm feeling high from alcohol or drugs I will drive a motor vehicle.
11. I tend to stumble when walking, or have more accidents than other people.
12. In any given week, I take at least one prescription drug without the recommendation of a physician (e.g., amphetamines, barbiturates).
13. I have problems with my sex life.
14. At least once during the week I will make bets for money.
15. After dinner I spend more time alone than talking with my family or friends.
16. I arrive at work late.
17. At least once during the week I have a shouting match with a coworker or supervisor.

THE URIC ACID HANDBOOK

Almost Always	Most of the Time	Some of the Time	Almost Never	Never
5	4	3	2	1
5	4	3	2	1
5	4	3	2	1
5	4	3	2	1
5	4	3	2	1
5	4	3	2	1
5	4	3	2	1
5	4	3	2	1
5	4	3	2	1
5	4	3	2	1
5	4	3	2	1
5	4	3	2	1
5	4	3	2	1
5	4	3	2	1
5	4	3	2	1
5	4	3	2	1
5	4	3	2	1

Behavioral indicators point total: _____

EMOTIONAL INDICATORS

Particulars
1. I have found the best way to deal with hassles and problems is to consciously avoid thinking or talking about them.
2. I have trouble remembering things.
3. I feel anxious or frightened about problems I can't really describe.
4. I worry a lot.
5. It is important for me not to show my emotions to my family.
6. It is hard for me to relax at home.
7. It's best if I don't tell even my closest friend how I'm really feeling.
8. I find it hard to talk when I get excited.
9. I feel very angry inside.
10. I have temper outbursts I can't control.
11. When people criticize me, even in a friendly, constructive way, I feel offended.
12. I feel extremely sensitive and irritable.
13. My emotions change unpredictably and without any apparent reason.
14. I feel like I really can't trust anyone.
15. I feel like other people don't understand me.
16. I really don't feel good about myself.
17. Generally, I am not optimistic about my future.
18. I feel very tired and disinterested in life.
19. Impulsive behavior has caused me problems.
20. I have felt so bad that I thought of hurting myself.

Almost Always	Most of the Time	Some of the Time	Almost Never	Never
5	4	3	2	1
5	4	3	2	1
5	4	3	2	1
5	4	3	2	1
5	4	3	2	1
5	4	3	2	1
5	4	3	2	1
5	4	3	2	1
5	4	3	2	1
5	4	3	2	1
5	4	3	2	1
5	4	3	2	1
5	4	3	2	1
5	4	3	2	1
5	4	3	2	1
5	4	3	2	1
5	4	3	2	1
5	4	3	2	1
5	4	3	2	1
5	4	3	2	1

Emotional indicators point total: _____

SLEEP INDICATORS

Particulars
1. I have trouble falling asleep.
2. I take pills to get to sleep.
3. I have nightmares or repeated bad dreams.
4. I wake up at least once in the middle of the night for no apparent reason.
5. No matter how much sleep I get, I wake up feeling tired.

PERSONAL HABITS

Particulars
1. I spend less than three hours a week working on a hobby of mine.
2. I spend less than one hour a week writing personal letters, writing in a diary, or writing creatively.
3. I spend less than 30 minutes a week talking casually with my neighbors.
4. I lack time to read the daily newspaper.
5. I watch television for entertainment more than one hour a day.
6. I drive in a motor vehicle faster than the speed limit for the excitement and challenge of it.
7. I spend less than 30 minutes a day working toward a life goal or ambition of mine.
8. My day-to-day living is not really affected by my religious beliefs or my philosophy of life.
9. When I feel stressed, it is difficult for me to plan time and activities to constructively release my stress.

Almost Always	Most of the Time	Some of the Time	Almost Never	Never
5	4	3	2	1
5	4	3	2	1
5	4	3	2	1
5	4	3	2	1
5	4	3	2	1

Sleep indicators point total: _____

Almost Always	Most of the Time	Some of the Time	Almost Never	Never
5	4	3	2	1
5	4	3	2	1
5	4	3	2	1
5	4	3	2	1
5	4	3	2	1
5	4	3	2	1
5	4	3	2	1
5	4	3	2	1
5	4	3	2	1

Personal habits point total: _____

No single question in this questionnaire proves you are experiencing stress, but by looking at the results of groups of questions, it may be possible to define what areas of your life stress affects the most. To determine these areas, add the circled numbers in each section and mark the point total for each section with an "X" on the appropriate dotted line below.

PERSONAL STRESS LEVELS

		Very Low	Medium	High	Very High	Danger
POINT TOTALS	Physical Indicators	22	30	38	48	54+
	Behavioral Indicators	18	27	36	45	50+
	Emotional Indicators	21	29	37	46	55+
	Sleep Indicators	5	8	10	12	14+
	Personal Habits	9	15	20	25	30+

Note the areas where you showed "very high" or "danger" levels of stress. These are problem areas you should focus on when you develop your Personal Stress Management Plan. If you have no point totals in the "very high" or "danger" zones, congratulations, you are doing a very good job of managing stress. In your Personal Stress Management Plan, focus on:

1. Building stress resources

2. Stress prevention through aerobic exercise, relaxation, nutrition, and sleep

EARLY WARNING SIGNS

On the lines below, write the three signs that occur earliest and most regularly when you're under stress. You may want to look back at your questionnaire to get an idea of what your early warning signs are. These signs give advance notice of being stressed and allow you to identify what causes you stress, and to take action before serious problems result.

1. _____

2. _____

3. _____

Date Questionnaire Completed: _____

(Keep this completed questionnaire for your future use. You can retake this questionnaire periodically and compare your results to keep track of your overall stress levels, pinpoint any new areas in your life that may be causing you stress, and track your progress of reducing previous stress-inducing areas of your life.)

CHAPTER 4

EAT RIGHT AND RECHARGE

High uric acid levels and joint pain can be controlled through a long-term disease management program. First, a lifestyle change is crucial to support the medical therapy suggested by your medical practitioner.

Here are two ways to manage your lifestyle, understand your body, and care for it:

- Understand that food *is* medicine. Watching what you eat and limiting your intake of high-fructose corn syrup, organ meats, red meat, fish, and alcoholic beverages can improve your body.
- Losing weight is a crucial part of your journey in managing high uric acid.

We will go deeper into these aspects of lifestyle change that can help reduce uric acid levels.

We understand that giving up the food you love is the hardest thing to do. Even when they make you feel rotten, comfort foods are tough to give up. What will life be like after they're gone? Will your new dietary restrictions drive your friends crazy? And what will you think of yourself if you fall off the wagon? The experience can be a bit of an emotional roller-coaster.

The key to parting amicably with a favorite food is minimizing your sense of deprivation. To this end, you must strive to open yourselves up to new food horizons as you replace old favorites. With this perspective in mind, let us explore specific and vital ways to drive a change in food habits.

BARRIERS TO CHANGING FOOD HABITS

A large mass of global consumers believe that maintaining a balanced diet is extremely important in contributing to their overall health. But consumers' personal definitions of health drive the fragmentation of diet beliefs and behaviors.

Recent popular diets, from keto to intermittent fasting and other such diet regimens, tell you to eat more protein, less sugar, or fewer and better carbs. However, what we've come to learn is that adopting and staying with diets like these can be extremely difficult.

Emotional attachments: Our connections with food, habits, or preferences may have deep cultural or emotional associations. For example, during your growing days, you may have been rewarded or comforted by being given particular food items by your loved ones or parents. As an adult, you may have treated yourself to special foods after achieving a milestone. Leaving behind the foods you associate with momentous life events is especially challenging.

The stress-relief effect: When you bite into that scrumptious, gooey piece of chocolate chip brownie (or any other guilty pleasure), you can sense your mood improving. That good feeling rarely lasts long, though. Biochemically, the body gravitates toward what makes it feel good at the moment, even if it's not serving you in the long term.

Habit: Even when a given food has a negative effect, you may be so used to the feeling that it seems normal. If you have been eating it daily, or even multiple times daily, you are habituated to how that food makes you feel. Avoiding it may make you unsettled until you start seeing the positive benefits of removing it from your diet.

Poor-me syndrome: You may worry that if you go without your favorite food, you'll be sentenced to bland, boring substitutes that are flat-out depressing to eat.

Fear of not fitting in: When you go out with your friends and see them ordering a plate of loaded nachos full of cheese and meat, you hardly want to be the person that asks for substitutes. It can make you feel self-conscious, and you may not want to be seen as a high-maintenance person who's difficult in restaurants, constantly checking ingredients and placing special orders.

SUGGESTED STRATEGIES FOR CHANGING FOOD HABITS

We firmly believe that it's crucial to applaud yourself when you make small wins in this journey to give up the food you love. So here are some ways that can help make this journey a wee bit easier.

Give up problem foods in stages: You may be better off taking a phased approach. For example, if you're eating dairy three times a day, try eating it twice a week, then once a day for another week, then every other day, and so on, until it's phased out entirely. Or, if you don't want to cut it out completely, gradually move to low-fat dairy.

Think of it as temporary: It may help to consider your abstinence as having a time limit, after which you might reintroduce the food into your diet on a limited basis to see how your body does.

Understand what you like about a specific food, then find it elsewhere: If you warmly associate chocolate cake with family, try making the pot roast you also loved as a kid. When you're craving something sweet, see if the candy-like sweetness of clementine makes you feel better than candy does.

Avoid equally harmful substitutes: Sometimes it can feel tempting to substitute certain items with slightly different ones to keep enjoying the taste of those products. However, they can be equally harmful in the long run and set you back in your journey of eating healthy.

Expand your palate: Start experimenting with new, high-quality whole foods. For example, try avocado on a sandwich instead of dairy-free cream cheese, or have your eggs with sweet potato instead of a gluten-free bagel.

Be patient: If you avoid bland substitutes and expand your palate, it generally takes two to four weeks for the changes in your diet to become established. Then, within a couple of months, you may be well past any cravings for the problem food.

Handle social situations tactfully: If you're feeling social pressure to eat/drink the thing you're giving up, don't make a big deal of your decision. Instead, you can say, "You know, I feel a lot better when I don't eat sugary stuff, so I'm cutting those foods out for a while to see how it goes without them."

Get professional support: A dietitian or nutritionist can help you understand your physical and emotional relationship to food, and they can be an ongoing source of support, suggesting foods you haven't tried and helping you assess the results.

FOOD AS MEDICINE

Food as medicine is a practice built on the knowledge that food and diet play important roles in disease prevention and management. Although credited for it, there is no evidence that Hippocrates stated, "Let thy food be thy medicine and thy medicine be thy food." However, in line with that philosophy, we are currently witnessing a reappraisal of the correlation between nutrition and pharmacology.

Recent studies not only underline the therapeutic potential of lifestyle interventions but also generate valuable insights into the complex and dynamic transition from health to disease.

There is no specific definition of the "food as medicine" concept. Still, it refers to making food and diet in an individual's health plan a crucial component, intending to prevent disease, reduce symptoms, or reverse a disease state. It is focused on the increased consumption of a variety of whole, minimally processed plant-based foods and limited intakes of highly processed foods rich in added sugar, oil, and salt.

Foods that proponents claim have medicinal properties, often due to supposed high levels of a particular micronutrient or biomolecule—sometimes referred to as functional foods—are of specific interest to people who consider food as medicine. A variety of herbs and spices, legumes, nuts and seeds, whole grains, and fruits and vegetables are known as functional foods. The bioactive compounds of plant-based functional foods are divided into six categories: flavonoids, phenolic acids, alkaloids, saponins, polysaccharides, and others. In addition, the mechanism by which these bioactive compounds exhibit a hypouricemic effect is summarized into three classes: inhibition of uric acid production, improved renal uric acid elimination, and improved intestinal uric acid secretion.

The "food as medicine" approach to health management challenges the construct of conventional medicine, which relies primarily on technological medical advancements to manage health and disease with pharmaceutical drugs.

BENEFITS OF THE FOOD AS MEDICINE APPROACH

Some benefits of a food as medicine health-care approach are:

Disease management: It is a part of evidence-based health practice that diet and food support the treatment of diseases. This demonstrates diet and nutrition's role in managing chronic disease. Improvements in diet quality can also reduce disease symptoms and improve quality of life.

Cost-effective: The prevalence of chronic diseases has increased worldwide, along with associated health-care costs. Using food as medicine could potentially reduce disease severity through better lab work, fewer medications, and fewer hospitalizations.

THE BOTTOM LINE

Can food be medicine? Food as medicine may be an emerging concept in the Western world, but many cultures around the globe have long recognized the role of diet in health. Healthy diets high in fruits, vegetables, whole grains, nuts and seeds, lean protein, and low-fat dairy could reduce the risk of chronic diseases, including heart disease and type 2 diabetes.

However, food as medicine is not a cure for all and should be used in conjunction with appropriate medical treatment.

DIET CAN HELP KEEP URIC ACID AT NORMAL LEVELS

Uric acid is excreted from the body after digestion of foods rich in purines, as explained in earlier chapters of this book.

People suffering from high uric acid levels must be extremely cautious of their diet and eating habits. Besides avoiding purine-rich food, you must avoid consuming too much fat, as it may reduce your body's ability to excrete uric acid.

Healthy eating and proper medication could help you maintain uric acid levels.

Following are some foods you must add to your diet to keep uric acid at normal levels:

Apples: Add apples to your life. Patients suffering from high uric acid get relief, as apples are enriched with malic acid and neutralize uric acid in the bloodstream.

Apple cider vinegar: People suffering from elevated uric acid levels can get relief by taking apple cider vinegar. You can add three teaspoons of vinegar to one glass of water. Have it two to three times every day to help treat high uric acid conditions.

Green bean juice: Extracted juice of green beans is an effective home remedy for treating gout. Consume this healthy juice twice daily to prevent high uric acid production in the blood.

Water: Water flushes out toxins from the body, including the excess presence of uric acid. So, having at least eight (8-ounce) glasses of water daily is recommended. Water plays a vital role in preventing gout attacks because it helps prevent the buildup of urate crystals. In addition, research has shown that exercise-induced sweating reduces uric acid excretion and increases uric acid levels in the body. This suggests dehydration can increase serum uric acid levels and is a risk factor for a gout attack.

In another study, adequate water consumption 24 hours before a gout flare-up was associated with a 46 percent decrease in recurrent gout attacks. Hence, if you or anyone you know is prone to high levels of uric acid, then place effort on remaining hydrated by drinking the optimal amount of water based on activity level. Uric acid cannot be diluted and efficiently released through the kidneys without water. The most important point to note is that dehydration also slows metabolism, leading to weight gain, which can cause or exacerbate gout.

Cherries: Cherries contain an anti-inflammatory substance called anthocyanin, which helps reduce uric acid levels. In addition, cherries prevent uric acid from crystallizing and getting deposited in the joints.

Berries: Berries, especially strawberries and blueberries, have enriched anti-inflammatory properties. Including them in your everyday diet helps prevent high uric acid levels in the blood. See Berries in a Gout Diet Plan on page 89.

Fresh vegetable juices: Carrot, beetroot, and cucumber juice are effective remedies to treat high uric acid in the blood.

Low-fat dairy products: High uric acid can also be treated by consuming low-fat dairy products. You can go for low-fat milk and yogurt/curd.

Lime: Lime juice contains citric acid, a solvent of uric acid. So, adding it to your daily diet helps prevent high uric acid levels. You could squeeze half a lime in a glass of water and have it every day or squeeze lime on your meal to make it tastier and healthier.

VITAMIN C-ENRICHED FOODS

Foods high in vitamin C disintegrate uric acid and flush it out of the body, which is an excellent way of treating elevated uric acid levels. Kiwi, gooseberry, guava, oranges, lemon, tomato, and other green leafy vegetables can be good sources of vitamin C.

Olive oil: Olive oil contains antioxidants and anti-inflammatory properties, so you can begin to cook your food in it. Cold-pressed olive oil is a good solution.

Celery seed: Celery seeds are a popular home remedy to treat high uric acid levels. Add them to your juices or soak them in water overnight before drinking.

High-fiber foods: Foods high in dietary fiber absorb uric acid from the bloodstream and help eliminate excess uric acid from your body through the kidneys. If you have been diagnosed with high uric acid, increase the consumption of dietary soluble fibers such as oats, apples, oranges, broccoli, pears, strawberries, blueberries, cucumbers, celery, carrots, and barley.

Green tea: Another way to treat high uric acid is by consuming green tea daily. This helps control hyperuricemia and lowers the risk of developing gout.

Tomatoes, cucumbers, and broccoli: Consumption of tomatoes, cucumbers, and broccoli before you start your meal is the best way to prevent the formation of high uric acid in your blood. In addition, their alkaline nature helps maintain uric acid in the bloodstream.

Omega-3: Add omega-3 fatty acids such as flax seeds and fish, including salmon, mackerel, herring, sardines, and walnuts, which help reduce swelling and inflammation.

THINGS TO AVOID

Sugary foods and beverages: While high uric acid is usually linked with a protein-rich diet, recent studies have shown that sugar can also be a potential cause. Most common are forms of added sugar, including table sugar and high fructose corn syrup. Fructose leads to high levels of uric acid. So don't forget to check food labels for sugar in all its forms when doing your grocery shopping. Eating more whole foods and fewer refined packaged foods reduces the intake of sugar.

Alcohol: When you consume alcohol, your trips to the bathroom increase, making you dehydrated and triggering high uric acid. This happens as your kidney is busy filtering out the products in the blood due to alcohol, instead of filtering uric acid and other wastes.

Manage your insulin levels: Too much insulin in the body can lead to high uric acid levels and weight gain. Therefore, it's best to check your insulin levels when you visit your doctor, even if you do not have diabetes mellitus.

We understand that maintaining a diet menu can be challenging and tricky. So here is an example of how you could plan yours.

A URIC ACID-FRIENDLY MENU FOR ONE WEEK

Eating a gout-friendly or hyperuricemia-friendly diet will help relieve pain and swelling while preventing future attacks. Here is a sample diet for a week.

Note on allergies: Please avoid all foods with which you may have faced allergies in the past. If you feel unusual symptoms after consuming the food item, do not go further with the diet, and discuss it with your medical advisor.

MONDAY

Breakfast: Smoothie with ½ cup blueberries, ½ cup spinach, ¼ cup Greek yogurt, and ¼ cup low-fat milk

Lunch: Quinoa salad with eggs and fresh sautéed vegetables

Dinner: Whole wheat pasta with chicken, spinach, bell peppers, and low-fat cheese

TUESDAY

Breakfast: Oats with yogurt and ¼ cup of berries (your choice)

Lunch: Whole grain sandwich with eggs and green salad

Dinner: Herb-baked salmon with cucumber and cherry tomatoes on the side

WEDNESDAY

Breakfast: Overnight oats made with ⅓ cup rolled oats, ¼ cup Greek yogurt, ⅓ cup low-fat milk, 1 tablespoon of chia seeds, ¼ cup assorted berries, and ¼ teaspoon of vanilla extract and refrigerated overnight

Lunch: Chickpeas, fresh vegetables, and chicken in a whole wheat wrap

Dinner: Stir-fried chicken and sautéed vegetables with brown rice

THURSDAY

Breakfast: Overnight chia seed pudding made with 2 tablespoons chia seeds, 1 cup Greek yogurt, and ½ teaspoon vanilla extract with sliced fruits of choice. Let sit in a bowl overnight/refrigerate if the temperature is warm.

Lunch: Salmon with a green salad

Dinner: Quinoa, spinach, eggplant, and feta salad

FRIDAY

Breakfast: French toast with strawberries or blueberries

Lunch: Whole grain bread toasted with boiled eggs and low-fat cheese with a green salad

Dinner: Stir-fried tofu and vegetables and/or chicken with brown rice

SATURDAY

Breakfast: Mushroom and zucchini frittata

Lunch: Stir-fried tofu and brown rice

Dinner: Homemade chicken burgers with a fresh green salad

SUNDAY

Breakfast: Two-egg omelet with spinach and mushrooms and/or tofu

THE URIC ACID HANDBOOK

Lunch: Chickpeas and fresh vegetables in a whole wheat tortilla

Dinner: Scrambled egg tacos made with scrambled eggs, spinach, and bell peppers in a whole wheat wrap

SOFT DRINK CONSUMPTION AND HYPERURICEMIA

People who frequently consume soft drinks are at increased risk of Hyperuricemia compared to their counterparts who "never" consume soft drinks.[23]

It has been reported that an intake of sugar-sweetened soft drinks was strongly related to the elevated risk of gout in men.[24]

COFFEE MAY REDUCE HYPERURICEMIA

Most scientific research studies suggest that coffee can play a role in lowering your risk of gout. Coffee contains various beneficial compounds, including minerals, polyphenols, and caffeine. Through several mechanisms, coffee is thought to reduce gout risk by lowering uric acid levels. Coffee may do this by increasing the rate at which your body excretes uric acid. Coffee is also thought to compete with the enzyme that breaks down purines in the body. This can lower the rate at which uric acid is created.

---

23 Joon Seob Lee et al., "Impact of Coffee / Green Tea/ Soft Drink Consumption on the Risk of Hyperuricemia: A Cross-Sectional Study," *International Journal of Environmental Research and Public Health* 18, no. 14 (2021): 7299, doi: 10.3390/ijerph18147299.

24 Hyon K. Choi and Cary Curhan, "Soft Drinks, Fructose Consumption, and the Risk if Gout in Men: Prospective Cohort Study," *British Medical Journal* 336, no. 7639 (2008): 309–312, doi: 10.1136/bmj.39449.819271.BE.

A recent review of the research found that drinking coffee was associated with lower levels of uric acid and fewer episodes of hyperuricemia in many cases. In one Japanese study, researchers found that coffee consumption had an inverse relationship with uric acid levels. Those who drank the most coffee (roughly 5 cups per day) had the lowest uric acid levels among the study participants. Although both coffee and tea were tested, these results seemed to apply only to coffee.[25]

This evidence implies that compounds in coffee other than caffeine may play a role in lowering uric acid levels.

WHY COFFEE

There are a few reasons why coffee may provide a protective effect against the buildup of uric acid. However, to understand why we first need to understand how certain medications for gout work.

Your doctor may prescribe two types of gout medication: xanthine oxidase inhibitors and uricosurics.

Xanthine oxidase inhibitors function by inhibiting the activity of xanthine oxidase. Xanthine oxidase is an enzyme that helps the body metabolize purines. Since purines are a source of uric acid, inhibiting this enzyme can help to keep uric acid levels low. Caffeine is considered to be a methyl xanthine.[26] Therefore, it can also compete with and potentially block the action of xanthine oxidase.

Uricosurics function by helping the kidneys rid the body of uric acid. Although caffeine isn't necessarily considered a uricosuric, it may function similarly. In addition, research has suggested that

---

25 Kiyohara et al., "Inverse Association between Coffee Drinking and Serum Uric Acid Concentrations in Middle-Aged Japanese Males," *British Journal of Nutrition* 82, no. 2 (August 1999), https://pubmed.ncbi.nlm.nih.gov/10743484.

26 Edward Roddy and Hyon Choi, "Epidemiology of Gout," *Rheumatic Diseases Clinics of North America* 40, no. 2 (2014): 155–175, DOI: 10.1016/j.rdc.2014.01.001.

THE URIC ACID HANDBOOK

chlorogenic acid,[27] a polyphenol found in coffee, may help to improve insulin sensitivity.

BERRIES IN A GOUT DIET PLAN

Berries are naturally low in purines. They are usually juicy, bright-colored fruit, a mix of sweet and sour. The ascorbic acid in berries may effectively repair cell damage caused by gout. In addition, all berries are high in flavonoids, which may possess potent anti-inflammatory and antioxidant properties.

The vitamin C in berries is required by the body to produce collagen, an essential component of connective tissue that may help repair damaged tissue in the body after a gout attack. Studies have also shown that it may effectively control uric acid in the body to help prevent urate crystal formation.

Blueberries, like all berries, are high in antioxidants that fight inflammation in the body. In addition, blueberry consumption seems to affect serum uric acid concentrations and their relationship with cardiovascular disease risk factors in a sex-specific manner. One cup of blueberries has 80 calories and no fat, providing a quarter of the daily vitamin C requirement.

Blackberries were used by the ancient Greeks as a natural remedy for gout and were known as "gout berry" many generations ago in American folk medicine. However, cherries were eventually discovered to be more effective since cherries contain an enzyme that may help neutralize uric acid.

---

27 Erick Prado de Olivira and Roberto Carlos Burini, "High Plasma Uric Acid Concentration: Causes and Consequences," *Diabetology and Metabolic Syndrome* 4, no. 4 (2012): 12, DOI: 10.1186/1758-5996-4-12.

Blackberries, though, outrank cherries in the antioxidant department, and remember that antioxidants are important because they neutralize the free radicals that may damage your tissues, usually in the big toe. Finally, they contain less sugar than many other fruits, making them better for your blood sugar levels and avoiding a significant release of insulin in the body. Finally, like all berries, blackberries may alkalize the body, though not as strongly as citrus fruits.

Strawberries are also high in antioxidants and vitamin C (90 mg per cup) but also contain high magnesium levels. This mineral may help reduce gout symptoms, including pain and swelling. One cup of strawberries provides you with 20 mg of magnesium, which is 5 percent of the daily recommended intake.

THE IMPORTANCE OF EATING ORGANICALLY GROWN BERRIES

Berries are notorious for being able to absorb high amounts of herbicides and pesticides. So people who suffer from gout should try to eat organically grown berries.

To ensure that the fruit you're eating is at its peak of freshness, look for locally grown organic berries or an organic pick-your-own berry farm near you. Ripe fruit also contains polyphenols and other beneficial compounds that aid gout treatment.

Freezing ripe berries is a simple approach to ensure that you have these "magic bullets" on hand when you need them.

However, they also contain oxalate, which may worsen gout in certain gout patients. This is derived from the chemical compound oxalic acid, and according to Columbia University researchers, a specific link exists between oxalate, uric acid, and kidney stones. So those with a history of kidney stones should seek medical advice before consuming strawberries in their diet since oxalate may aggravate the symptoms of gout but, more importantly, may increase the risk of certain gout patients developing kidney stones.[28]

Also, note that more than 90 percent of strawberries consist of water, and gout sufferers need plenty of water in their diet to get rid of urate crystals in the body. Americans eat an average of three-and-a-half pounds of fresh strawberries each year. Every state in the US and province in Canada grows strawberries in the summertime, so try to eat locally grown organic ones, if possible.

Raspberries may fight inflammation in gout the same way aspirin and ibuprofen do by shutting off signals sent by COX-1s and COX-2s enzymes responsible for the body's inflammatory response. There are only 64 calories in 1 cup of strawberries; it is cholesterol-free and contains 186 mg of potassium, which is very important for gout sufferers. Drinking tea made from red raspberries or their leaves is also very effective in treating gout pain, according to several gout sufferers.

NUTRIENTS THAT HELP LOWER URIC ACID

Vitamin C helps the kidneys cleanse waste materials (such as uric acid), boost the production of red blood cells, and reduce the risk of kidney stones because of its antioxidant characteristics.

Vitamin A's antioxidant properties are required for cellular growth, which improves the kidneys' ability to remove excess fats, salts, sugars, and uric acid from the blood. Fruits high in vitamin A, like

---

28 https://pubmed.ncbi.nlm.nih.gov/19779706.

vitamin C, can help relieve gout symptoms and improve kidney function.

Potassium is a mineral that also serves as an electrolyte. In gout, an excess of salt in the system is connected to the production of uric acid. Salt also makes it more difficult for the kidneys to eliminate other waste products, such as uric acid. As a result, most gout sufferers try to keep their salt intake to a minimum.

Potassium is often underestimated in maintaining good kidney functions, yet it plays a critical role in eliminating excess salt from the body.

Magnesium is a mineral that is required for a variety of bodily processes. First, magnesium is essential for gout patients who want to reduce their uric acid production. Second, it makes toxins more soluble, making it easier for them to filter out via the kidneys and the bladder. Finally, magnesium-rich fruits can help the kidneys and relieve gout symptoms.

FRUIT FOR THOUGHT

Almost all fruits are alkaline forming, even if they are acidic when raw. This means that alkaline by-products form after fruits are ingested and metabolized. Urine becomes less acidic as a result. The kidneys may transfer more uric acid to the bladder and urine because uric acid is more soluble in alkaline solutions.

The correct fruits in your diet can help your kidneys function properly and flush out more uric acid, which is essential to keeping your gout symptoms in check.

Keep pushing and attempting more natural gout treatments if you want long-term, permanent relief from the agony of gout.

After an understanding of how to make changes to our diet plan so that uric acid is lowered, let us dive into the next major change in our lifestyle, which is really a humongous challenge for most people: losing weight!

WEIGHT LOSS AND URIC ACID

Losing weight can potentially reduce a person's average serum uric acid levels. We can say this with some degree of confidence because clinicians have proven that weight loss achieved from bariatric surgery and dietary changes resulted in positive outcomes for people at risk of gout or with elevated uric acid levels. Being overweight, especially if that extra weight is in our bellies, is often linked to elevated levels of uric acid because excessive fat leads to insulin resistance, making our body less efficient at removing uric acid.

Here is a surprise for all who are desperate to lose weight: getting more sleep can help you lose weight, as can an exercise plan. However, a question that may often arise is whether we should walk or engage in any exercise when we have gout, which is a manifestation of elevated uric acid.

Here we attempt to answer this predicament.

First, if you are going through a gout flare-up, then, under the advice of a clinician and a physical therapist, you should consider adding different heart-pumping activities into your exercise routine, such as swimming or riding a stationary bike. Both are especially good options for gout patients because they don't put as much pressure on the weight-bearing joints of the feet, ankles, and knees while helping us keep our weight in check.

WHY DO WALKING AND EXERCISE MATTER WHEN WE HAVE GOUT?

If left untreated, gout can erode and destroy our joints. So while it's important to follow our medication treatment plan as advised by our clinicians, keeping our joints healthy when we have gout should also involve physical activity and exercise for two main reasons:

- Maintaining a healthy weight prevents excessive weight-bearing force on our joints. Coincidentally, a healthy diet to control weight, such as the DASH (Dietary Approaches to Stop Hypertension) diet designed to reduce high blood pressure, has been found to help people reduce their uric acid levels as well. However, we should be careful not to lose weight too quickly, as this sudden weight loss can raise uric acid.

- Exercising helps control gout by lowering uric acid levels to prevent gout attacks. Researchers have found that fat in the body carries more uric acid than muscles. Thus, when we reduce body fat, we can reduce uric acid levels in our blood. Building cardiovascular health through exercise is also very important for people with gout because they have a higher risk of developing high blood pressure. Gout is also strongly associated with developing coronary artery disease.

CHAPTER 5

THE FOOD FESTIVAL

We all hate diet plans, don't we?

Why would you want to plan every part of your meal and hold back when the aroma of food is so tempting? So here is a way to change your outlook on what you eat. If you were to have a food festival, wouldn't you plan the menu? Think of this journey as a food festival. Yes, you heard it right, you will have a 28-day food festival and enjoy each bit of it. What's more, you can include others in this journey, too.

This chapter includes a mix of suggestions from low-fructose foods, the DASH diet,[29] and a low-purine diet. DASH stands for dietary approaches to stop hypertension. The DASH diet is a healthy-eating plan designed to help treat or prevent high blood pressure (hypertension). The DASH diet includes foods that are rich in potassium, calcium, and magnesium. These nutrients help control blood pressure. The diet limits foods that are high in sodium, saturated fat, and added sugars. A low purine diet will typically center around fruits, vegetables, and whole grains. The diet will minimize the consumption of red meat, seafood, and alcohol.

Earlier in this book, you learned what foods to avoid and what foods can heal the problem of elevated uric acid. Keep in mind, however, that just knowing the good and the harmful food items for this type of condition is inadequate for you to make the change. Rather, a complete lifestyle change is required, which may often entail a

---

29 Mayo Clinic Staff, "DASH Diet: Tips for Dining Out," MayoClinic.org, June 25, 2021, https://www.mayoclinic.org/healthy-lifestyle/nutrition-and-healthy -eating/in-depth/dash-diet/art-20044759.

change in lifestyle for your partner and caregiver and maybe the entire family. So, if this is reality, let's try to make it fun!

A well-stocked kitchen will ensure you eat smart and have the right foods to create delicious meals that are gout friendly, friendly for elevated uric acid levels, and super healthy. Our definition of well stocked is a bit different in this case. It does not mean big quantities of all foods, it means stocking up with the right type of foods and NOT stocking the wrong type, as initially, we all tend to crave our comfort foods and may fall off the track.

Do go back to the foods that are the best for you or your loved one and make a list that can be ready on your phone for when you go grocery shopping. Please note that some canned foods are higher in sodium, especially soups, tomato products, and vegetables. The Nutrition Facts label is your best guide for keeping a aware of the brands of canned foods that make sense for you and your family. Choose foods that have less than 10 percent of the daily value in sodium. Rinsing some foods can help remove some sodium, but purchase "no salt added" or low sodium if you can. Lowering sodium in your diet helps lower blood pressure and protect the kidneys, which work hard to eliminate uric acid.

Here is a list that will be handy for you to stock your pantry.

CANNED FOODS

- Artichoke hearts packed in water
- Beans, low-sodium, canned
- Broth, low-sodium: chicken or vegetable (less than 140 mg of sodium per 8-ounce serving)
- Salmon, pouch, or low-sodium, canned
- Tomato products, no-salt-added

CONDIMENTS, OILS, VINEGAR

- Hot sauce: Louisiana-style, Frank's RedHot
- Mustard: Chinese hot, Dijon, or dried
- Oil: chili, extra-virgin olive, light olive, sesame
- Soy sauce, low-sodium
- Sriracha
- Vinegar: apple cider, balsamic, red wine, rice

BEVERAGES

- Tart cherry juice
- Water: plain bottled, naturally flavored seltzer

GRAINS AND LEGUMES

- Pearl barley
- Whole grain bread and hamburger rolls
- Whole wheat breadcrumbs
- Whole wheat flour
- Lentils, dried
- Oats: old-fashioned rolled, steel-cut
- Whole wheat pasta,
- Rice: brown, wild
- Tortillas: corn, whole wheat

NUTS, SEEDS, AND DRIED FRUIT

- Dried fruit: apples, cherries, cranberries, raisins
- Unsalted nuts: walnuts, pine nuts
- Nut butter: unsalted, all-natural
- Seeds: chia, flax, sesame

SPICES AND SWEETENERS

- Black pepper
- Capers
- Cayenne pepper
- Chili powder
- Cilantro, fresh
- Cinnamon, ground
- Coriander, ground
- Cream of tartar
- Cumin, ground
- Curry powder
- Dill
- Extract: almond, vanilla

- Garlic powder
- Ginger, fresh
- Honey
- Italian seasoning
- Maple syrup, pure
- Mrs. Dash, any blend you prefer, or other salt-free seasonings
- Oregano
- Red pepper flakes
- Rosemary
- Sage
- Salt: kosher and sea
- Sugar: brown, granulated
- Tarragon
- Thyme
- Fresh or ground turmeric
- Unsweetened cocoa powder

It may be a great idea to go to an Asian store and buy some of these spices fresh to grind/dry at home and keep ready for use on your kitchen counter.

REFRIGERATOR STOCKING GUIDE

Low-fat dairy helps reduce uric acid levels, so we suggest that you keep your refrigerator well stocked with items that are low-fat. If you have dairy allergies, there are a variety of milk substitutes commercially available.

DAIRY, EGGS, AND DAIRY SUBSTITUTES

- Cheese: blue, feta, Monterey Jack, mozzarella, Parmesan, pepper jack
- Eggs
- Greek yogurt, plain, low-fat
- Milk, low-fat
- Orange juice
- Tofu, extra-firm

FRUITS AND VEGETABLES

- Avocado
- Bell peppers
- Cherries, in season
- Citrus: lemons, limes, oranges
- Garlic

- Green vegetables: bok choy, broccoli, kale, spinach, Swiss chard
- Onions: shallots, scallions
- Pomegranate
- Sweet potatoes

BEEF, PORK, FISH, POULTRY

- Canadian bacon
- Fish: cod, flounder, haddock, halibut, salmon (wild or farmed)
- Pork tenderloin
- Poultry: low-fat cuts such as skinless chicken or turkey breast; ground turkey; turkey sausage
- Red meat: lean cuts such as flank, tenderloin, or sirloin

We understand that you are a busy person with a lot to handle through the day and cannot afford to be off schedule. Having a well-stocked freezer as a backup to those hectic days when you cannot stop at the grocery store is a lifesaver!

You may ask, are frozen fruits and vegetables as healthy as fresh ones? Yes, they are! Frozen may even surpass the nutritional quality of fresh ones.

Just-picked, farm-fresh produce is loaded with nutrition and should be your first choice. But the longer produce is in transit or stays on the supermarket shelf, the more nutrients are lost. Once fruits and vegetables are picked, they sit in a warehouse before they are hauled into a truck to be delivered to a grocery store and then finally make it into your refrigerator.

Conversely, when fruits and veggies are harvested for commercial freezing, they are picked when fully ripe—at their nutritional peak. So, if you can't eat just-picked produce, frozen is the next best thing.

Here is a list of recommended foods to freeze:

- Berries: blackberries, blueberries, cherries, strawberries
- Fish: see the refrigerator stocking guide

- Frozen yogurt, low-fat
- Lean red meats: see the refrigerator stocking guide
- Whole grain pancakes or waffles

Before you get the chef's cap on to enjoy the food festival, let us remind you of some essential things you need in your kitchen.

COOKING EQUIPMENT GUIDE

Don't worry about getting yourself fancy kitchen gadgets to start the food festival. Having the fundamentals on hand works just fine. Some tools speed up the preparation process, and the quicker, the better for our hectic lives. Isn't it?

We understand that a lack of counter or storage space and the high cost of specific items can be a dampener. And there's nothing wrong with cooking the old-fashioned way.

ESSENTIALS

- 9-inch square baking pan
- 10- or 12-inch nonstick skillet
- 12-cup muffin tin
- Baking sheet
- Blender
- Grater
- Pots, assorted sizes
- Saucepan
- Slow cooker

MEASURING

- Liquid measuring cup
- Set of dry measuring cups
- Set of measuring spoons

MIXING AND CUTTING

- Knives: chef's, paring
- Mixing bowls: small, medium, and large

- Silicone scraper
- Spatula

- Whisk
- Wooden spoon

MISCELLANEOUS
- Mason jars, small
- Parchment paper
- Ramekins

- Vegetable peeler
- Wooden skewers
- Zester

GOOD TO HAVE
- Apple peeler and corer
- Citrus juicer
- Food processor

- Indoor or outdoor grill
- Stovetop grill pan

Before we spell out the appropriate recipes for your elevated uric acid levels, we would like you to understand that you do not have to do this alone; on the contrary, we would like you to have this food festival with your family and friends. What's more, we would encourage you to use these recipes even when you throw a party. So eat like the rest of your family; just don't overindulge.

PEC MEAL PLAN

To make PEC your new mantra, all you need to do is make sensible decisions about eating!

To do so, follow the PEC formula:

Pay attention to portion sizes
Eat fewer processed foods or fast foods
Choose healthy foods

Our endeavor through this chapter is to share with you recipes that help you to go **PEC**. So, we will follow the PEC formula to create the food festival. Whether you are a pro in the kitchen or are just learning your way around, you can make these recipes. Tips are included to offer to simplify, modify, or diversify a recipe. We have also included some nutritional education regarding these recipes.

A delicious PEC meal doesn't have to break the bank. These simple recipes are made of inexpensive ingredients and can be cooked within 30 minutes, from start to finish. Treat yourself to scrumptious dishes that are easy to make and yummy to eat. You deserve it!

We suggest you make a four-week PEC meal plan as a starting point. You can choose things to make from the recipes in the breakfast, lunch, and dinner categories later in the chapter. Don't forget to put certain items in the snacks and desserts category for everyday. You may ditch snacks and desserts on those days when you can resist the temptation.

Here is a one-week meal plan template you can use.

	Breakfast	Lunch	Dinner	Snack/Dessert
Monday				
Tuesday				
Wednesday				

	Breakfast	Lunch	Dinner	Snack/Dessert
Thursday				
Friday				
Saturday				
Sunday				

Congratulations on starting the food festival!

BEYOND THE NORMAL

We understand that there will be days that will be beyond normal. On those days, you will be fighting hard to hold back and may find yourself declining invitations to birthday parties, anniversary celebrations, and other such occasions just so that you can keep to your PEC Meal Plan.

But we surely do not want you to feel socially isolated; we would love for you to carry the spirit of the food festival well into your socializing. Just remember PEC, and your life will be sorted.

Keeping your focus on PEC will help you to:

- Be mindful. Pay attention to what you are eating. Get a sense of when you are starving and listen to your body.
- Eat a small meal or snack before the party so you are not hungry at the party.
- Enjoy some small portions of the special foods, and eat slowly.
- Fill your plate with DASH-friendly vegetables.
- Stay hydrated with seltzer water with vitamin C–rich lemon or lime juice.

Most of all, focus on enjoying conversations and having a good time rather than eating.

WHEN YOU ARE EATING AT A RESTAURANT

It's a great feeling to go to a unique cuisine restaurant and have someone else do the cooking for you. Isn't it? But since you are on a PEC Meal Plan, be prepared before you walk into the restaurant.

You can go online and view the menu beforehand so that you are making PEC decisions about your order at the restaurant. When at the restaurant, ask your server specific questions regarding the ingredients; they are well trained to accommodate inquiries and special requests per your requirement.

If you are going to have a late night, have a small snack or a meal in advance so that you are not starved, as that may lead to wrong desperate decisions, and you may fall off your PEC Meal Plan. Be mindful of your alcohol intake. And limit sodium intake. Listen to your body; if necessary, eat a PEC portion of the meal and pack the rest for others to eat at home.

We know that restaurant meals differ, and it can be challenging to decide on an order while following a PEC meal plan. So here are some strategies to try and keep to your PEC meal plan.

ASIAN FOOD

Turn away from: fried foods or spareribs, fried egg rolls, Peking ravioli, dim sum, pot stickers, soy sauce, and teriyaki sauce.

PEC MEAL CHOICES

- Steamed entrées, vegetables, tofu
- Rice (brown preferred), plain noodles, lettuce roll-ups
- Request that your food be prepared without soy sauce, fish sauce, or MSG; all are high in sodium

ITALIAN CUISINE

Turn away from: alfredo, bolognese, or carbonara sauce; buttered garlic bread; and creamy salad dressings.

Have small portions of clam or mussel dishes.

Use grated cheese in moderation.

PEC MEAL CHOICES

- Plain pasta (e.g., spaghetti, fettuccine, penne, tortellini, ravioli)
- Breadsticks; bread with extra-virgin olive oil
- Wine sauces (e.g., marsala)
- Mixed-greens salad with oil and vinegar or vinaigrette dressing

MEXICAN FOOD

Turn away from: sour cream; fried entrées or sides; green chili (if cream-based); and fried taco shells.

Limit red meat to 6-ounce servings (e.g., enchiladas filled with minced beef/meat) and watch the amount of cheese used.

PEC MEAL CHOICES
- Baked, broiled, grilled, or steamed chicken or fish dishes preferred
- Plain rice (brown preferred); soft tacos; burritos; fajitas
- Salsa (no cream); avocado; guacamole

BARBECUE

Turn away from: barbecue sauce, steak sauce, horseradish, sausage, hot dogs, cornbread, MSG, or teriyaki sauce.

Limit red meats (grilled or broiled) and seafood (shrimp, lobster) to 6 ounces; pulled meats (pork, beef, and chicken) are high in sodium, so consider sharing a meal.

PEC MEAL CHOICES
- Grilled or broiled chicken or fish; 2-inch square of cornbread; grilled vegetables
- Marinades with wine, lemon juice, oil, vinegar, garlic, honey, herbs, and spices

BUFFETS

Turn away from: red meats and seafood (shrimp, lobster, sardines) or limit them to a 6-ounce serving.

- Soups (high in sodium); olives; pickles; bacon bits; salted nuts; croutons; olive salads; macaroni salad; relishes; pickles

- Entrées or vegetables in creamed or cheese sauces (escalloped, au gratin)
- Fried foods
- Marinated meats
- Creamy salad dressings or sour cream

PEC MEAL CHOICES
- Grilled, sautéed, or broiled fish or chicken
- Roasted, steamed, or grilled vegetables
- Salad bar, coleslaw, gelatin salads, cottage cheese, oil and vinegar or vinaigrette dressing

DESSERT

Turn away from: dough piecrusts; milk chocolate; coconut; cheesecake; custard; puddings; ice cream; and gelato.

PEC MEAL CHOICES

All fresh fruit or canned, unsweetened fruit; sugar cookies; angel food cake; gelatin; low-fat frozen yogurt or low-fat ice cream; puddings with low-fat milk; graham crackers; cobblers or crisps; graham cracker pie crusts; dark chocolate squares

* * *

Note: These strategies can be beneficial when you are on a well-deserved vacation, too. Don't let vacay time lead you to a health crisis; it should only leave you with beautiful memories, so remember the PEC Meal Plan choices and focus on the scenery you see.

In the next section of this chapter, we will help you customize the PEC Meal Plan for yourself. The recipes are divided into categories that will make your choice easier.

CHAPTER 6

BREAKFAST RECIPES

As you are well aware, breakfast is the first meal of the day, usually eaten in the morning. It refers to **breaking the fasting period of the previous night.** Since it is about breaking the fast, it becomes a crucial meal, replenishing your supply of glucose to boost your energy levels and alertness while providing other essential nutrients required for good health.

Many studies have shown the health benefits of eating breakfast. It improves your energy levels and ability to concentrate in the short term and can help with better weight management and reduced risk of type 2 diabetes and heart disease.

Many people skip it for various reasons like rushed schedules and laziness in cooking a meal. There are plenty of ways to make it easier to fit breakfast into your day while ensuring that it is sumptuous and fun.

WHY WE THINK BREAKFAST IS SO IMPORTANT FOR YOU

When you wake up, you may not have eaten for up to 10 hours. Breakfast replenishes the stores of energy and nutrients in your body. It is that time of the day when specific things are required, like an up in energy levels.

The body's energy source is glucose. Glucose is broken down and absorbed from the carbohydrates you eat. The body stores most of its energy as fat. But your body also stores some glucose as glycogen, most of it in your liver, with smaller amounts in your muscles. During times of not eating, the liver breaks down glycogen and releases it into your bloodstream as glucose to keep your blood sugar levels stable. This is especially important for your brain, which relies almost entirely on glucose for energy. Eating breakfast boosts your energy levels and restores your glycogen levels to keep your metabolism up for the day.

Skipping breakfast may seem like an excellent way to reduce overall energy intake. However, with a higher energy intake, breakfast eaters tend to be more physically active in the morning than those who don't eat until later in the day.

Breakfast allows your body to take in essential vitamins, minerals, and nutrients. Foods we eat for breakfast are generally rich in folate, calcium, iron, B vitamins, and fiber. In fact, people who eat breakfast are more likely to meet their recommended daily intake of vitamins and minerals.

People who regularly eat breakfast **are less likely to be overweight or obese.** It is thought that eating breakfast may help you control your weight because:

- It prevents large fluctuations in your blood glucose levels.
- Breakfast fills you up before you become really hungry, so you're less likely to just grab whatever foods are nearby when hunger strikes (for example, high-energy, high-fat foods with added sugars or salt).
- Breakfast boosts brainpower.

If you don't have breakfast, you might find yourself a bit sluggish and struggling to focus. Often if you miss breakfast, by the time your next meal time comes up, you may be starving, so your PEC Meal choice may go for a toss. Those who eat breakfast generally have more healthy diets overall, have better eating habits, and are less likely to be hungry for snacks during the day than people who skip breakfast.

People who skip breakfast tend to nibble on snacks during the midmorning or afternoon. This can be a problem if those snacks are low in fiber, vitamins, and minerals but high in fat and salt. Basically, they may not be according to your PEC Meal Plan. Without the extra energy that breakfast can offer, some people feel lethargic and turn to high-energy foods and drinks to get them through the day.

Some common reasons for skipping breakfast include:

- Not having enough time or wanting to spend the extra time in bed
- Trying to lose weight
- Being too tired to bother
- Being bored of the same breakfast foods
- Not feeling hungry in the morning
- Having no breakfast foods readily available in the house
- Avoiding the cost of buying breakfast foods

While skipping breakfast is not recommended, good nutrition is not just about the number of meals you have each day. If you don't have breakfast, aim to make up for the nutritional content you missed at breakfast with your lunch and dinner.

IDEAS FOR HEALTHY BREAKFAST FOODS

Research has shown that schoolchildren are more likely to eat breakfast if easy-to-prepare breakfast foods are readily available at home. Some quick suggestions include:

- Porridge made from rolled oats. When choosing quick oats, go for the plain variety and add your own fruit afterward as the flavored varieties tend to have a lot of added sugar.
- Whole grain cereal (such as untoasted muesli, bran cereals, or whole wheat biscuits) with milk, natural yogurt, and fresh fruit

- Fresh fruits and raw nuts
- Whole meal, whole grain, or sourdough toast, or English muffins or crumpets with baked beans, poached or boiled eggs, tomatoes, mushrooms, spinach, salmon, cheese, avocado, or a couple of teaspoons of spreads such as hummus or 100 percent nut pastes (such as peanut or almond butter)
- Smoothies made from fresh fruit or vegetables, natural yogurt, and milk
- Natural yogurt with some fresh fruit added for extra sweetness and some raw nuts for crunchiness
- If you're low on time, you can still have breakfast

Early starts, long commutes, and busy morning schedules mean many of us don't make time to sit down to breakfast before heading out for the day. Whatever your reason for being time-poor in the morning, there are still ways that you can fit in a PEC breakfast.

Some quick ideas that can help you gather yourself for a PEC breakfast:

- Prepare some quick and healthy breakfast foods the night before or on the weekend, such as zucchini bread, healthy muffins, or overnight oats (to make, soak rolled oats in milk overnight in the fridge, and add fruit/nuts to serve). A preprepared breakfast means you can grab it and eat it at home, on the way to work, or at your destination.
- Keep some breakfast foods at work (if allowed) to enjoy once you arrive.
- Get in the habit of setting your alarm for 10 to 15 minutes earlier than usual to give yourself time to have breakfast at home.

- Swap out any time-wasting habits in the morning (such as checking your emails or scrolling social media), and use this time for breakfast instead.

- Prepare for the next day the night before to free up time in the morning to have breakfast.

If it's still hard for you to eat food first thing in the morning, we have some suggestions.

- Eat smaller portions in the night or evening.

- Find new recipes and ingredients for different types of foods to increase your breakfast appetite, make it more exciting for yourself.

- Create a PEC breakfast plan, which makes you look forward to the next day's plan.

It's often hard to think up what to plan for specific meals, and more so when keeping in mind to avoid some types of food. We understand it well and have tried to make it easy for you to use this section of the book for ready recipes that will help you be mindful of the specifics. In a while you will get used to planning your meals and may not need the guide any further. Happy cooking!

CHERRY OR BERRY SMOOTHIE

Weekday breakfast can be quick and easy with smoothies. Toss the ingredients into a blender, and it's done. This smoothie includes the option of turmeric, which reduces inflammation. Leftovers can be stored in the fridge for about three days. Just blend again before serving.

Serves: 2 | Prep time: 5 minutes

1½ cups frozen pitted cherries or any other berries

2 cups low-fat or nondairy milk, such as unsweetened almond milk or soy milk

1 tablespoon chia seeds

½ teaspoon grated peeled fresh ginger or turmeric

½ cup crushed ice

1. In a blender, combine all ingredients. Blend until smooth.

2. Modify every day by replacing the cherries with available berries or soft pulpy fruits like peaches.

TIP: If you have a sweet tooth, you can add 1 tablespoon of honey to your smoothie.

PINEAPPLE-GRAPEFRUIT SMOOTHIE

Serves: 1 | Prep time: 15 minutes

1 cup chopped pineapple

½ grapefruit

1 banana

5 ounces water

½ cup cilantro

½ cucumber

2 tablespoons chia seeds

1. Place all the ingredients into a blender and process until smooth.

2. Pour into a glass and serve.

CHIA SEED PUDDING

You can prepare the chia seeds the previous night

Serves: 2 | Prep time: 15 minutes plus overnight to set

2 tablespoons chia seeds

¾ cup water

fresh fruits or dry fruits

2 tablespoons nuts

2 to 3 pieces dry figs, chopped

1 tablespoon sunflower seeds

1 cup low-fat plain yogurt

1. Soak the chia seeds in the water in a bowl, and let sit for 15 minutes. The consistency will change to a jelly-like formation. Now place the bowl in the refrigerator for the night.

2. In the morning, add the fresh or dry fruits, nuts, chopped figs, and sunflower seeds to the chia seeds in the bowl. Mix it in with a spoon.

3. Add the low-fat yogurt and serve in two bowls.

HONEY ORANGE POMEGRANATE YOGURT

You may buy pomegranate seeds, or if you have a whole pomegranate, cut it in half and tap the outer shell to remove seeds. You can do this the night before or on the weekend to avoid delays in the morning.

Serves: 2 | Prep time: 15 minutes

1 cup plain low-fat Greek yogurt

zest of ½ orange

juice of ½ orange

1 tablespoon honey

½ teaspoon grated fresh ginger or turmeric

½ cup pomegranate seeds

1. Stir together the yogurt, orange zest and juice, honey, and ginger in a bowl. Serve with the pomegranate seeds sprinkled on top.

TIP: If you are allergic to oranges, you can replace the orange juice and zest with any other chopped soft fruit. Pineapple goes well in this recipe, too.

SPICED APPLE WALNUT OVERNIGHT OATS

This is a grab-and-go breakfast option to serve chilled. Don't use instant oats, which are too mushy. Instead of cinnamon, try pumpkin pie spice, ginger, or nutmeg for a different flavor on different days.

Serves: 1 | Prep time: 5 minutes plus overnight to rest

½ cup low-fat or nondairy unsweetened milk, such as almond or rice milk

¼ cup plain low-fat Greek yogurt

½ cup rolled oats

¼ cup fresh or dried apples or any other dried fruits, such as apricots

2 tablespoons chopped walnuts

2 teaspoons chia seeds

½ teaspoon ground cinnamon

1 tablespoon honey

1. Combine all ingredients except for the honey. If you are using fresh fruits instead of dried ones, add them in the morning. Mix well in a mason jar or a small Tupperware container that is easy to carry. Cover and refrigerate overnight.

2. In the morning, stir to your consistency of choice. If you don't prefer cold oats, heat them in the microwave for 1 minute on high power. Drizzle honey on top and it's ready to carry to work.

TIP: For a twist, try topping the overnight oats with nut butter or stir in some pumpkin purée before eating.

OMELET AND BELL PEPPER

Omelets are easy to customize to satisfy your tastes. Using bell pepper can add vitamin C to your breakfast. You can refrigerate leftovers for up to five days and reheat in the microwave for about one minute on high power.

Serves: 2 | Prep time: 10 minutes | Cook time: 15 minutes

1 tablespoon extra-virgin olive oil

1 red bell pepper, seeded and sliced

1 clove garlic, minced

2 large eggs

4 large egg whites

¼ teaspoon freshly ground black pepper

¼ teaspoon sea salt

¼ cup shredded Monterey Jack cheese

1. Brush a nonstick skillet with the olive oil and place on the stovetop over medium heat. Wait for the oil to bubble up, then add the red bell pepper and cook for about 5 minutes, stirring occasionally, until soft and slightly brown.

2. Add the garlic and cook for a few seconds, stirring to combine. Arrange the red bell peppers and garlic at the base of the pan in a single layer. Reduce the heat to low.

3. Whisk the eggs, egg whites, pepper, and salt together in a bowl. Pour the mixture over the red bell pepper and garlic layer. Let it settle and cook. The eggs will settle around the bell pepper layer. Do not stir. Cover the skillet for a few seconds. The egg will no longer stick to the skillet when done.

4. Using a spatula, pull the edges of the omelet away from the sides of the pan, tilt the pan, and let the uncooked eggs flow in case there is any underneath.

5. Cook until the eggs are set, 1 to 2 minutes), then sprinkle the cheese over the eggs. Turn off the heat.

6. Using a spatula, fold the omelet. Let sit, covered, until the cheese melts, about 1 minute.

TIP: Season with black pepper or oregano to serve. To store the omelet in the refrigerator, set it aside to cool and place it in an airtight container.

SALMON AND KALE SCRAMBLE

*Salmon has remarkable anti-inflammatory properties,
as it is loaded with omega-3 fatty acids.*

Serves: 4 | Prep time: 10 minutes | Cook time: 15 minutes

1 tablespoon extra-virgin olive oil	2 large eggs
1 shallot, minced	6 large egg whites
2 cups chopped stemmed kale	¼ teaspoon freshly ground black pepper
1 (5-ounce) pouch wild-caught salmon	1 teaspoon dried dill

1. In a large skillet over medium to high heat, heat the olive oil until it shimmers.

2. Add the shallot and kale. Cook, stirring occasionally until the vegetables are soft. The shallot will turn somewhat transparent within a few minutes.

3. Add the salmon. Cook, stirring, for 1 minute more. Reduce the heat to medium.

4. Whisk the egg yolks, egg whites, pepper, and dill in a bowl and add the eggs to the vegetables. Cook for about 4 minutes, stirring occasionally until the eggs are set.

TIP: Add all the ingredients you love to the scrambled eggs. Garlic, onions, mushrooms—use your imagination and stay in the PEC meal zone. The salmon can be replaced by any low-sodium, low-fat meat you prefer, like turkey sausage. You can replace the kale with vegetables like asparagus, spinach, or chopped bell pepper.

CHAPTER 7

LUNCH AND DINNER RECIPES

You can plan a PEC meal by fixing a salad, sandwich, or soup for lunch. You can freeze your soup and carry it to work or pack a salad that is relatively easy to put together. Here are some recipes for healthy and satisfying meals.

TUSCAN BEAN, KALE, AND TURKEY SAUSAGE SOUP

This is a soup that the whole family will enjoy.

Serves: 4 | Prep time: 10 minutes | Cook time: 25 minutes

1 tablespoon extra-virgin olive oil

8 ounces Italian turkey sausage

1 medium onion, chopped

1 red bell pepper, seeded and chopped

2 cups chopped stemmed kale

6 to 7 cloves garlic, minced

1 (15.5-ounce) can low-sodium white beans (such as cannellini), drained and rinsed

1 teaspoon dried Italian seasoning

1 (14-ounce) can no-salt-added diced tomatoes, with its juice

4 cups low-sodium chicken broth or vegetable broth

¼ teaspoon freshly ground black pepper

pinch red pepper flakes

1. Heat the olive oil in a large pot over medium-high heat until it shimmers. Add the turkey sausage and cook for about 5 minutes, stirring and crumbling with a spoon, until it turns brown.

2. Add the onion, red bell pepper, and kale and cook for 5 minutes, stirring.

3. Add the garlic and cook for 30 seconds, stirring constantly.

4. Add the white beans, Italian seasoning, tomatoes and their juice, chicken or vegetable broth, black pepper, and red pepper flakes. Bring to a simmer and reduce the heat. Cook for another 5 minutes, stirring occasionally, until the soup is a bit thick.

5. Freeze the soup to store and transport, or refrigerate for up to 5 days. Use microwavable containers for easy meals. Reheat on the stovetop or in the microwave.

CHICKEN NOODLE SOUP WITH SNAP BEANS

Serves: 4 | Prep time: 10 minutes | Cook time: 20 minutes

2 tablespoons extra-virgin olive oil

1 onion, chopped

8 ounces boneless, skinless chicken tenders, cut into 1-inch pieces

1 carrot, chopped

1 pound snap beans

1 stalk celery, chopped

4 cloves garlic, minced

5 cups low-sodium broth of choice

2 teaspoons dried rosemary

juice of 1 lemon

¼ teaspoon sea salt

¼ teaspoon freshly ground black pepper

1 (14-ounce) packet rice noodles

1. Heat the olive oil in a large pan over medium heat until it shimmers. Add the onion and chicken. Cook for about 5 minutes, stirring occasionally, until opaque. 2. Add the carrot, beans, and celery. Cook for about 5 minutes more, stirring until the vegetables begin to soften.

2. Add the garlic. Cook for 30 seconds, stirring constantly.

3. Stir in the broth, rosemary, lemon juice, salt, and pepper. Bring to a simmer.

4. In a separate pot, bring the rice noodles to a boil until they turn transparent and soft (may take 7 to 10 minutes). Add the noodles to the soup pan and let them cook together for 5 minutes. It's ready to be served!

KALE, WALNUT, AND STRAWBERRY SALAD WITH CITRUS VINAIGRETTE

This salad makes a great light lunch, snack, or side. Using baby spinach instead of kale keeps the greens bite-size. Both spinach and strawberries are anti-inflammatory and excellent sources of vitamin C. This can serve as a complete meal for the family or a start to the meal.

Serves: 2 | Prep time: 10 minutes

For the Salad:

4 cups fresh kale

1 cup sliced fresh strawberries

1 cup sliced cherry tomatoes

½ cup chopped walnuts

¼ cup citrus vinaigrette

For the Citrus Vinaigrette (makes 1½ cups):

1 small shallot, finely chopped

¾ cup olive oil

¼ cup champagne vinegar or white wine vinegar

3 tablespoons fresh lemon juice

2 tablespoons fresh orange juice

¼ teaspoon finely grated lemon zest

Kosher salt and freshly ground black pepper, to taste

1. In a large bowl, combine the kale, strawberries, cherry tomatoes, walnuts.

2. Combine all of the vinaigrette ingredients except the salt and pepper in a small jar.

3. Season vinaigrette to taste with salt and pepper. Shake to blend.

4. Add vinaigrette to the salad and toss!

TIP: If storing this salad or carrying it out, do not mix the salad and vinaigrette until just before eating, or the kale will lose water. You can also omit the vinaigrette and season this salad simply with 1 tablespoon each of extra-virgin olive oil and vinegar.

TIP: Vinaigrette can be made 1 week ahead. Cover and store in the refrigerator. Shake before using.

SALMON AND ARUGULA SALAD WITH BLACKBERRY VINAIGRETTE

This is an excellent salad to use up any leftover cooked fish, including whitefish or shellfish such as shrimp. You can also use low-fat, low-sodium meat such as chicken or turkey.

Serves: 2 | Prep time: 10 minutes

For the Salad:

4 cups baby arugula

5 ounces cooked wild-caught salmon, flaked

2 scallions, white and green parts, finely chopped

¼ cup blackberry vinaigrette

For the Blackberry Vinaigrette (makes 1½ cups):

¼ cup red wine vinegar

1 teaspoon low-carb sweetener

1 tablespoon Dijon mustard

½ teaspoon onion powder

½ cup fresh blackberries (substitute with blueberries if needed)

¼ cup olive oil

kosher salt and pepper, to taste

1. In a large bowl, combine the arugula, salmon, and scallions.

2. Combine all vinaigrette ingredients except salt and pepper in a small jar.

3. Season vinaigrette to taste with salt and pepper, then shake to thoroughly mix. Refrigerate for up to a week and use when required.

4. Add ¼ cup of vinaigrette to the salad, then toss.

ITALIAN SALAD

Feel free to add fresh chopped veggies to up the salad's nutrition. To avoid the extra salt, use additional chicken as a substitute for bacon.

Serves: 4 | Prep time: 10 minutes

1 cup chopped boneless skinless chicken breast, sautéed

3 ounces bacon, chopped

2 cups cherry tomatoes, halved

1 (14-ounce) can no-salt-added artichoke bottoms, halved

½ cup or 2 ounces shredded mozzarella cheese

1 cucumber, chopped

¼ cup fresh basil leaves

¼ cup pine nuts

¼ cup plain low-fat Greek yogurt

¼ cup apple cider vinegar

1 clove garlic, minced

½ teaspoon freshly ground black pepper

4 to 5 mint leaves

1. In a large salad bowl, combine the chicken, bacon, tomatoes, artichokes, cheese, cucumber, basil, and pine nuts.

2. In another bowl, whisk the yogurt, vinegar, garlic, and pepper together.

3. Add the dressing to the chicken, bacon, and vegetables. Toss to combine.

4. Garnish with mint leaves.

CURRIED LENTILS

Serves: 4 | Prep time: 10 minutes | Cook time: 30 minutes

2 tablespoons extra-virgin olive oil

1 onion, chopped

2 carrots, chopped

1 red bell pepper, seeded and chopped

3 cloves garlic, minced

2 tablespoons curry powder

1 teaspoon ground turmeric

¼ teaspoon sea salt

4 cups low-sodium vegetable broth

1½ cups dried lentils

¼ cup light coconut milk (optional)

1. Heat the olive oil in a large pot over medium heat until it shimmers, for about 1 minute.

2. Add the onion, carrots, and red bell pepper. Cook for about 5 minutes, stirring until the vegetables begin to soften and the onions turn transparent.

3. Add the garlic, curry powder, turmeric, and salt. Cook for 1 minute and keep stirring.

4. Stir in the vegetable broth and lentils. Bring to a boil. Reduce the heat to medium. Simmer, uncovered, for about 20 minutes, stirring occasionally until the lentils reach your desired texture. They should be squeezable in between your fingers.

TIP: If you prefer a creamier curry, stir in up to ¼ cup light coconut milk before serving.

TIP: Serve with a bowl of cooked brown rice or quinoa. This recipe freezes well; you can store it in the refrigerator in a ready-to-carry Tupperware container along with the rice or quinoa.

VEGETABLE AND TOFU STIR-FRY

Stir fries are versatile, quick, and accessible. Add your favorite vegetables; you can grab some prechopped vegetables from the grocery's produce section or opt for a bag of mixed frozen peppers.

Serves: 4 | Prep time: 10 minutes | Cook time: 15 minutes

2 tablespoons extra-virgin olive oil

6 scallions, white and green parts, chopped

1 red bell pepper, seeded and sliced

1 green bell pepper, seeded and sliced

1 orange bell pepper, seeded and sliced

1 head broccoli, cut into 5 to 6 pieces

2 carrots, chopped

12 ounces extra-firm tofu, patted dry and cut into ½-inch pieces

2 tablespoons Low-Sodium Ginger Stir-Fry Sauce

For the Low-Sodium Ginger Stir-Fry Sauce:

1½ cups chicken stock (or Broth)

1 tablespoon corn starch (if you're looking for a healthier options, swap for tapioca flour or arrowroot powder)

¼ cup reduced-sodium soy sauce

1 teaspoon honey

1 tablespoon sesame oil

½ cup rice vinegar

1 inch fresh ginger (you can use powdered ginger)

1. Heat the olive oil in a large skillet over medium heat for 1 minute, or until it shimmers.

2. Add the scallions, red, green, and orange bell peppers, broccoli, carrots, tofu, and any other vegetable you like. Cook for 5 to 7 minutes, stirring until the vegetables begin to soften. If the vegetables seem too stiff even after 7 minutes, add a dash of salt and cover the skillet with a lid.

3. Add all ingredients for the Low-Sodium Ginger Stir-Fry Sauce to a small pot. Stir together on low heat for 3 to 4 minutes, or until it thickens, and the sauce is ready.

4. Pour stir-fry sauce into the skillet. Continue cooking and stirring until the sauce thickens a bit. This should take about 2 minutes.

TIP: If you need the ginger stir-fry sauce to be gluten-free, swap the soy sauce for tamari.

TIP: The stir-fry freezes well—for up to 6 months—or will keep refrigerated for up to 5 days. Serve with brown rice or a portion of quinoa.

WHITE BEAN CHILI

This chili goes well with brown rice/quinoa or whole wheat tortillas. Feel free to use red beans instead of white.

Serves: 4 | Prep time: 10 minutes | Cook time: 20 minutes

2 tablespoons extra-virgin olive oil

1 red onion, finely chopped

1 red bell pepper, finely chopped

3 cloves garlic, minced

1 teaspoon ginger paste

1 (15.5-ounce) can low-sodium white beans, drained and rinsed

2 cups low-sodium vegetable broth or water

2 tablespoons chili powder

½ teaspoon sea salt

½ teaspoon dried oregano

1 teaspoon ground cumin

pinch cayenne pepper

1 avocado, peeled, pitted, and chopped

1. Heat the olive oil in a pot over medium heat for 1 minute until it shimmers.

2. Add the red onion and red bell pepper. Cook for 5 to 7 minutes, stirring until the vegetables soften.

3. Add the minced garlic and ginger paste. Cook for 30 seconds, stirring constantly.

4. Add white beans, vegetable broth, chili powder, sea salt, oregano, cumin, and cayenne pepper. Bring to a boil. Reduce the heat to medium and simmer, stirring occasionally, for 5 minutes.

5. Serve topped with chopped avocado. Garnish with up to 1 tablespoon per serving of low-fat sour cream or plain yogurt and low-sodium salsa.

TIP: The curry freezes well. Make a double batch and freeze for up to 6 months or refrigerate for up to 5 days. Reheat on the stovetop or in the microwave.

LENTIL BARLEY STEW

This stew is a complete meal. Replace the barley with farro if you prefer that texture.

Serves: 4 | Prep time: 10 minutes| Cook time: 40 minutes

2 tablespoons extra-virgin olive oil

1 yellow onion, chopped

2 carrots, chopped

2 celery stalks, chopped

1 garlic clove, minced	1 bay leaf
6 cups low-sodium vegetable broth	1 tablespoon dried thyme
1 (15.5-ounce) can of no-salt-added crushed tomatoes, drained	1 teaspoon ground turmeric
	¼ teaspoon freshly ground black pepper
1 cup pearl barley	1 tablespoon cornstarch
1 cup dried lentils	1 tablespoon water

1. Heat the olive oil on a skillet over medium to medium heat until it shimmers, about 1 minute

2. Add the onion, carrots, and celery. Cook for about 5 minutes, stirring, until the vegetables begin to soften and the onion turns transparent.

3. Add the garlic. Cook for 30 seconds.

4. Stir in the vegetable broth, tomatoes, barley, lentils, bay leaf, thyme, turmeric, and pepper, and bring to a boil. Reduce the heat to medium-low. Simmer for about 25 minutes, stirring frequently, until the barley and lentils are soft. Remove and discard the bay leaf.

5. In another bowl, whisk the cornstarch and water until smooth. Stir this into the stew and cook for a few minutes until the stew starts to thicken. Don't forget to stir.

Variation with rice: If you want to make it gluten-free, replace the barley with 1 cup of brown rice instead of the barley. Then, add the lentils and cook for 25 minutes more until the rice and lentils are tender. Alternatively, omit the barley and stir in cooked brown rice just before serving.

TIP: If you make a double batch and have a lot of leftovers, this freezes well for up to 6 months, or it keeps refrigerated for about 5 days.

RED BEANS AND BROWN RICE

Red beans and rice is a flavorful and traditional Cajun combination that tastes good with sausages. This vegan version has the same great Cajun flavors but without the meat.

Serves: 4 | Prep time: 10 minutes | Cook time: 15 minutes

2 tablespoons extra-virgin olive oil

1 yellow onion, chopped

1 green bell pepper, seeded and chopped

1 celery stalk, chopped

½ cup low-sodium vegetable broth

1 (15.5-ounce) can low-sodium kidney beans, rinsed and drained

2 cups cooked brown rice

1 teaspoon garlic powder

1 teaspoon dried thyme

½ teaspoon dried oregano

pinch red pepper flakes

½ teaspoon freshly ground black pepper

2 teaspoons Louisiana hot sauce

1. Heat the olive oil in a large pot on medium heat until it shimmers, 1 minute.

2. Add the onion, green bell pepper, and celery, and cook for about 5 minutes, stirring all the while.

3. Add the vegetable broth, kidney beans, brown rice, garlic powder, thyme, oregano, red pepper flakes, black pepper, and hot sauce. Bring to a simmer. Cook for 5 minutes, stirring until warmed through.

TIP: If you have a spicy taste palate add ¼ teaspoon of cayenne pepper. It's best to start with a pinch, taste, and add a little more to reach your desired spice levels.

BALSAMIC CHICKEN BREAST WITH BRUSSELS SPROUTS

Serves: 4 | Prep time: 10 minutes | Cook time: 30 minutes

3 tablespoons extra-virgin olive oil, divided

4 (3-ounce) pieces of boneless chicken breast, pounded

½ teaspoon sea salt, divided

¼ teaspoon freshly ground black pepper

2 cups Brussels sprouts, ends removed and leaves separated

½ cup aged balsamic vinegar

pinch red pepper flakes

1. Heat 1½ teaspoons of olive oil in a large nonstick skillet over medium-high heat until it shimmers, about 1 minute.

2. Season the chicken with the salt and pepper. One at a time, cook the chicken pieces for about 3 minutes per side until cooked through, adding 1½ teaspoons of olive oil for each. Set the chicken aside, tented with aluminum foil.

3. Add the remaining 1 tablespoon of olive oil to the pan and heat until it shimmers. Add the Brussels sprouts and the remaining ¼ teaspoon of salt. Cook for about 3 minutes until the sprouts soften. If you like your Brussels sprouts browned, cook them for an additional 15 minutes, stirring occasionally, or until they reach your desired level.

4. Add balsamic vinegar and bring to a simmer. Add the chicken and turn it in the sprouts and vinegar several times to coat. Serve the chicken with the sprouts spooned over the top.

TIP: As an alternative, roast the Brussels sprouts separately from the chicken. Preheat the oven to 400°F. Trim the ends off the sprouts and halve them. Place them in a single layer, cut side down on a rimmed baking sheet, and drizzle with 1 tablespoon of olive oil. Roast for 45 to 50 minutes or until browned.

After cooking the chicken in the skillet, add the balsamic vinegar and red pepper flakes and bring to a simmer. Simmer for about 5 minutes until reduced by half. Turn each piece of chicken in the warm balsamic vinegar to coat it. Serve the warmed balsamic vinegar spooned over the chicken and Brussels sprouts.

TIP: To make the Brussels sprouts, trim the ends and separate the leaves from the heads, which will happen naturally once the ends are cut. This trick substantially decreases the time it takes to cook Brussels sprouts.

TURKEY WITH WILD RICE AND SPINACH

The cooked wild rice in this recipe is an excellent source of vitamin B6 and magnesium, and it adds nice flavor and texture.

Serves: 4 | Prep time: 10 minutes | Cook time: 20 minutes

2 tablespoons extra-virgin olive oil

12 ounces 93% lean ground turkey breast

2 cups chopped stemmed spinach

1 red onion, chopped

juice of 1 lemon

1 teaspoon ground turmeric

½ teaspoon sea salt

2 cups cooked wild rice

2 cloves garlic, minced

1. Heat the olive oil in a nonstick skillet until it shimmers, about 1 minute.

2. Add the ground turkey breast and cook for about 5 minutes, stirring and crumbling with a spoon, until it starts to brown.

3. Add the spinach. Cook for about 5 minutes more, until the spinach softens. 4. Add the red onion, lemon juice, turmeric, salt, and wild rice. Cook for 5 minutes, stirring occasionally.

4. Add the garlic. Cook for 30 seconds and continue stirring.

TIP: Wild rice takes about 45 minutes to cook; plan ahead to make this meal come together quickly. Cooking a batch and freezing it in 1-cup servings can save you time for weekday meals. Thaw it in the refrigerator or microwave before adding it to this dish.

ASIAN TURKEY AND CHINESE CABBAGE STIR-FRY

Serve this recipe with ½ cup brown rice or quinoa.

Serves: 4 | Prep time: 10 minutes | Cook time: 15 minutes

2 tablespoons extra-virgin olive oil

12 ounces 99% extra-lean ground turkey breast

6 scallions, white and green parts, sliced, plus more for garnishing

3 cups chopped Chinese cabbage, cut into bite-size pieces (If you can get baby ones for this dish, all you need to do is halve it lengthwise to prep it.)

2 tablespoons Stir-Fry Sauce (see page 124 for recipe)

2 tablespoons sesame seeds, toasted

1. Heat the olive oil in a large nonstick skillet over medium-high heat until it shimmers, 1 minute.

2. Add the ground turkey breast. Cook for about 5 minutes, stirring and crumbling with a spoon.

3. Add the scallions and Chinese cabbage and cook for about 3 minutes, stirring until the vegetables soften.

4. Add the stir-fry sauce. Cook for about 2 minutes more, until it thickens. Garnish with sesame seeds and additional scallions.

SPAGHETTI WITH MEATBALLS TOMATO SAUCE

Serves: 4 | Prep time: 15 minutes | Cook time: 35 minutes

½ cup whole-grain bread crumbs

½ cup low-fat milk or dairy substitute

12 ounces chicken breast

½ onion, finely chopped

1 large egg, beaten

1 teaspoon dried Italian seasoning

1 teaspoon garlic powder

½ teaspoon sea salt

⅛ teaspoon freshly ground black pepper

pinch red pepper flakes

2 tablespoons extra-virgin olive oil

1 can low-sodium tomato puree

4 ounces whole wheat spaghetti, cooked according to the package instructions and drained

1. In a large bowl, stir together the bread crumbs and milk. Let sit for 10 to 15 minutes. To this mixture, add the chicken breast, onion, egg, Italian seasoning, garlic powder, salt, black pepper, and red pepper flakes, and mix to combine. Form the mixture into meatballs.

2. Heat the olive oil in a nonstick skillet over medium-high heat until it shimmers, 1 minute.

3. Work in batches and cook the meatballs for about 15 minutes, turning only occasionally, until they are cooked.

4. Add the tomato puree to the meatballs and bring to a simmer. Simmer for about 5 minutes, turning the meatballs to coat. Spoon the meatballs and sauce over the spaghetti.

Gluten-free option: you can choose gluten-free spaghetti or make zucchini noodles using a spiralizer or by peeling the zucchini into strips with a vegetable peeler and using a sharp knife to cut the strips into noodles. Use gluten-free bread crumbs for the meatballs, too.

PESTO CHICKEN WITH ROASTED TOMATOES

Serve with whole wheat pasta, brown rice, or baked sweet potatoes. Use any leftover chicken in salads for lunches or reheat in the microwave for a delicious meal in a hurry.

Serves: 4 | Prep time: 10 minutes | Cook time: 1 hour

3 cups cherry tomatoes, halved

4 boneless, skinless chicken thighs or breasts

1 to 2 tablespoons pesto sauce

1. Preheat the oven to 375°F.

2. Spread the cherry tomatoes in an even layer on the bottom of a rimmed baking dish. Top them with the chicken thighs. Spoon some of the pesto over the top of each chicken piece. Bake for about 1 hour, until the chicken juices run clear.

TIP: If you are using skinless thighs or breasts, it's a good idea to toss the tomatoes with 2 tablespoons of extra-virgin olive oil before adding them to the pan.

CHICKEN SATAY WITH PEANUT SAUCE

It's straightforward to make homemade peanut sauce, which is delicious on this chicken satay or with other meats as well. Serve the chicken with a salad and brown rice to complete the meal. While most chicken satay comes grilled on skewers, it's just as easy here to bake it without the skewers—and it makes it easier to eat, too.

Serves: 4 | Prep time: 15 minutes, plus 4 hours to marinate | Cook time: 10 minutes

For the Satay:

2 tablespoons low-sodium soy sauce

juice of 2 limes

4 to 5 cloves garlic, minced

1 tablespoon grated peeled fresh ginger

½ teaspoon ground coriander

12 ounces boneless chicken breast, cut into ½-inch strips

For the Peanut Sauce:

6 scallions, white and green parts, finely chopped

½ cup no-salt-added all-natural peanut butter

¼ cup low-fat coconut milk

2 tablespoons fresh cilantro leaves

1 clove garlic, minced

1 tablespoon low-sodium soy sauce

2 teaspoons freshly squeezed lime juice

1 teaspoon grated peeled fresh ginger

1 teaspoon sesame oil

pinch red pepper flakes

To make the Satay:

1. Use a blender to combine the soy sauce, lime juice, garlic, ginger, and coriander. Blend until smooth and pour into a zip-top bag. Add the chicken, seal the bag, and refrigerate to marinate for 4 hours.

2. Preheat the broiler to its highest setting and set an oven rack in its most elevated position. Remove the chicken from the marinade and place it on a broiler pan. Broil for 5 to 7 minutes, until the chicken juices run clear.

To make the Peanut Sauce:

1. In a blender or food processor, combine the scallions, peanut butter, coconut milk, cilantro, garlic, soy sauce, lime juice, ginger, sesame oil, and red pepper flakes. Blend until smooth. Spoon the peanut sauce over the chicken satay and serve.

TIP: If you want to grill the satay, soak wooden skewers in water while you marinate the chicken. Thread the chicken onto the skewers. Preheat the grill to high and brush it with oil. Grill the skewers for about 2 to 3 minutes per side and serve with the peanut sauce.

SOUTHWESTERN BOWL

What's nice about this dish is how quickly the bowls come together and how easy they are to customize with whatever you have available in your fridge.

Serves: 4 | Prep time: 15 minutes, plus 4 hours to marinate | Cook time: 10 minutes

juice of 2 limes

6 scallions, white and green parts, roughly chopped

¼ cup fresh cilantro leaves

2 cloves garlic, minced

1 teaspoon chili powder

½ teaspoon sea salt

3 tablespoons extra-virgin olive oil, divided

12 ounces boneless chicken breast, cut into ½-inch strips

2 cups cooked brown rice

1 avocado, peeled, pitted, and chopped

1 tomato, chopped

¼ cup plain low-fat Greek yogurt

1. Use a food processor to combine the lime juice, scallions, cilantro, garlic, chili powder, salt, and 2 tablespoons of olive oil. Process until smooth.

2. Reserve 2 tablespoons of the marinade and pour the rest into a zip-top bag. Add the chicken to it and seal the bag. Refrigerate to marinate for at least 4 hours.

3. Heat the olive oil in a large nonstick skillet over medium-high heat until it shimmers, 1 minute

4. Remove the chicken from the marinade and pat it dry. Add it to the hot oil and cook for 5 to 7 minutes. Add the reserved marinade. Cook for 1 minute more.

5. To assemble the bowls, place ½ cup of rice into each bowl. Top each bowl with the chicken, chopped avocado, chopped tomato, and a dollop of yogurt.

PORK CHOPS WITH GINGERED APPLE SAUCE

If you are too busy and have no time to make fresh applesauce, stir 1 tablespoon of grated peeled fresh ginger into store-bought unsweetened apple sauce.

Serves: 4 | Prep time: 10 minutes | Cook time: 20 to 30 minutes

4 sweet-tart apples, peeled, cored, and chopped

¾ cup water

2 tablespoons light brown sugar

1 tablespoon grated peeled fresh ginger or 1 teaspoon ground ginger

1 teaspoon dried thyme

½ teaspoon sea salt

¼ teaspoon freshly ground black pepper

4 thin-cut pork chops, trimmed of excess fat

2 tablespoons extra-virgin olive oil

1. In a large pot, combine the apples, water, brown sugar, and ginger. Cover the pot and cook for 15 to 20 minutes, until the apples are soft.

2. In a small bowl, stir together the thyme, salt, and pepper. Sprinkle this seasoning on the pork chops.

3. Heat the olive oil in a large skillet over medium-high heat until it shimmers, and add the pork chops. Cook for about 3 minutes per side, until golden brown.

4. Spoon the apple sauce over the pork chops to serve.

MEAT LOAF MUFFINS

Making meatloaf muffins means the meatloaf cooks much more quickly than a whole loaf. Serve with steamed veggies, such as green beans, brown rice, or roasted baby potatoes.

Serves: 6 | Prep time: 10 minutes | Cook time: 30 minutes

½ cup whole wheat breadcrumbs

½ cup low-fat milk or milk substitute

9 ounces 95% extra-lean ground beef

9 ounces 93% lean ground turkey

2 tablespoons Dijon mustard

2 carrots, grated

½ red onion, finely chopped

1 tablespoon dried thyme

1 teaspoon garlic powder

¼ teaspoon sea salt

¼ teaspoon freshly ground black pepper

1. Preheat the oven to 350°F.

2. In a large bowl, combine the bread crumbs and milk. Let sit for 5 minutes, then add the ground beef, ground turkey, mustard, carrots, red onion, thyme, garlic powder, salt, and pepper to the bread crumb mixture. Mix well.

3. Press the meat mixture into a 12-cup muffin tin, filling the wells.

4. Bake for 25 to 30 minutes, until the internal temperature reaches 160°F.

TIP: These freeze well in zip-top bags for up to 6 months. Thaw in the fridge and reheat in the microwave.

CHAPTER 8

DESSERT RECIPES

CHOCOLATE ALMOND MERINGUE COOKIES

These cookies are easy to make, but they take awhile to bake. But the light, crispy, chocolatey cookies are tasty and satisfying. For best results, use an egg beater or stand mixer to get the right texture on the meringue.

Makes: 18 cookies | Prep time: 15 minutes | Cook time: 25 minutes

3 large egg whites

⅛ teaspoon cream of tartar

pinch of salt

½ teaspoon almond extract

⅔ cup sugar

1 tablespoon unsweetened cocoa powder

1. Preheat the oven to 300°F. Line a baking sheet with parchment paper. Set aside.

2. In a bowl, use a handheld electric mixer to combine the egg whites, cream of tartar, salt, and almond extract. Beat until foamy.

3. While still beating, 1 tablespoon at a time, add the sugar. Continue to beat for about 7 minutes, until stiff peaks form. Gently fold in the cocoa powder. Spoon the meringue, in 18 portions, onto the prepared baking sheet.

4. Bake for 20 to 25 minutes, until the cookies are crisp.

OATMEAL AND DRIED CRANBERRY COOKIES

Cranberries are rich in antioxidants, and oats contain heart-healthy soluble fiber. These oatmeal cookies do include butter, so if you need to watch saturated fat in your diet, pay attention to the serving size noted so you can maintain a PEC meal plan.

Makes: 12 cookies | Prep time: 15 minutes | Cook time: 10 minutes

1⅓ cups old-fashioned rolled oats

⅓ cup flax seeds

⅓ cup all-purpose flour

1 teaspoon ground cinnamon

½ teaspoon ground ginger

¼ teaspoon baking soda

¼ teaspoon baking powder

pinch of salt

zest of 1 orange

6 tablespoons unsalted butter, at room temperature

¾ cup packed light brown sugar

1 teaspoon vanilla extract

1 large egg, beaten

¾ cup dried cranberries

1. Preheat the oven to 350°F. Line a baking sheet with parchment paper. Set aside.

2. In a medium bowl, whisk the oats, flaxseed, flour, cinnamon, ginger, baking soda, baking powder, salt, and orange zest. Set aside.

3. In a large bowl, cream together the butter, brown sugar, and vanilla. Stir in the egg. Add the dry ingredients to the wet ingredients, stirring until well combined. Drop in 12 spoonfuls onto the prepared baking sheet.

4. Bake for 8 to 10 minutes, until the cookies are browned.

TIP: These freeze well, so you can have cookies throughout the week. You can also freeze the dough in single cookies before baking, store them in zip-top bags, and bake one at a time so you can have a warm, fresh cookie to satisfy that sweet tooth.

HONEY LEMON CHIA PUDDING WITH BERRIES

Chia seeds, when soaked overnight, thicken and become gelatinous, so they make an easy and tasty, no-cook pudding. Sprinkle with fresh berries of your choice when ready to serve.

Serves: 4 | Prep time: 10 minutes, plus overnight to chill

6 tablespoons chia seeds

2 cups low-fat milk or milk substitute

2 tablespoons honey

zest of 1 lemon

1 cup fresh berries of choice

1. In a medium bowl, whisk the chia seeds, milk, honey, and lemon zest. Pour the mixture into 4 (4-ounce) dessert bowls. Cover with plastic wrap and refrigerate overnight. Serve with ¼ cup of berries of your choice or the ones readily available as a topping over each pudding cup.

TIP: Adjust the thickness of this pudding by adding more liquid (for a thinner consistency) or more chia seeds (for a thicker consistency). About 30 minutes before serving, check the pudding to see how the texture is. If it is too thin, add 1 teaspoon of chia seeds and let sit for 30 minutes more. If it's too thick, stir in 1 teaspoon of milk at a time until you reach the desired consistency.

BAKED APPLES

Baked apples taste best in the fall when they are in season.
Choose a sweet-tart apple for the best flavor and texture.
Serve with a scoop of low-fat frozen vanilla yogurt or mix
1 tablespoon of pure maple syrup and ¼ cup plain low-fat
Greek yogurt and spoon over the top of the warm apples.

Serves: 4 | Prep time: 10 minutes | Cook time: 30 minutes

4 apples	½ teaspoon ground cinnamon
¼ cup packed light brown sugar	4 teaspoons unsalted butter
½ teaspoon ground ginger	4 tablespoons chopped walnuts

1. Preheat the oven to 350°F.

2. To prepare the apples, slice off the top (about ¼ inch) from each apple. Using a spoon or knife, cut out the core, leaving the bottom intact so it forms a bowl.

3. Place the apples, cut side up, in a small baking dish. In a small bowl, stir together the brown sugar, ginger, and cinnamon. Spoon the mixture into the center of each apple.

4. Top the brown sugar mixture with 1 teaspoon of butter per apple. Sprinkle the walnuts on top. Bake for about 30 minutes, until the apples are tender.

OVERCOMING ELEVATED URIC ACID: WALK THE TALK

We began this journey with an understanding that trying to overcome the obstacle of elevated uric acid levels is daunting. This unnerving challenge is not unmanageable if you decide to nip it in the bud.

Being conscious of the consequences of not dealing with elevated levels of uric acid can be the first step. As you may have already gathered, this issue creeps into our lives specifically when we experience unmanaged stress levels coupled with lifestyle issues that lead us to being unmindful about the food we eat, or the quantities that we take in.

WHY DO WE NEED TO KEEP URIC ACID IN CHECK?

Too much or too little of anything is not acceptable. Nature designed everything to be finely balanced. So is the case with uric acid! The levels of uric acid in blood plasma should be in the range of 3.5 to 4.5 mg/dl at the lower level and 7 to 8 milligrams per deciliter (mg/dl) at the highest level for men, and 2.5 to 3.5 mg/dl at the lowest level and 6 to 7 mg/dl at the highest level for women.

Not dealing with an elevated level of uric acid can lead to ailments that are life impeding. This kind of condition can lead to disruptions in day-to-day activities and the development of long-term chronic health concerns like permanent bone, joint, and tissue damage; kidney disease; and heart disease if left untreated. High uric acid levels and type 2 diabetes, high blood pressure, fatty liver disease, and Alzheimer's disease are closely connected.

This is the primary reason you and your family should focus on treating elevated uric acid early, before it can cause any serious problems like gout, kidney disease, or heart disease.

WHAT DO WE NEED TO DO TO KEEP URIC ACID IN CHECK?

The first and foremost thing to do is keep a lookout for certain symptoms that indicate that the uric acid levels may be affected.

Some of the signs and symptoms that you should look out for:

1. Joint pain. Gout affects your joints. Some of the commonly affected joints include ankles, knees, elbows, wrists, and fingers.

2. A lingering discomfort after the initial pain subsides. It can last for a few weeks or longer.

3. Difficulty moving your joints.

4. Swollen, tender, and red joints.

If these symptoms arise, it's advisable to reach out to a physician and check out the implications. Simultaneously, keep a watch on your meal routine and exercise levels. Don't miss out on the Stress Indicators Questionnaire (see page 65).

Following a routine that includes medication, allopathic or alternate, is vital if uric acid levels are found to be elevated.

HOW DO WE REORGANIZE OURSELVES TO MANAGE URIC ACID LEVELS?

1. Regularly check stress levels by maintaining a document that notes certain regular patterns, as shown on page 75 of this book.

2. Plan your yoga routine so that you are in rhythm with yourself and your body.

3. Maintain a meal plan with the help of the PEC strategy suggested on page 101.

4. Regularly consume food that's low in purines and plan restaurant meals as mentioned earlier in this book.

5. If medicines are prescribed, it's important to be regular and consistent with the medication and adhere to the complete dosage.

6. Use the ready recipes so that the process of cooking a special meal doesn't become a burden.

7. Keep up your spirits and optimism, as you are not at a point of no return. Remember, this is treatable and very much in your control!

ABOUT THE AUTHORS

Urvashi Guha is a cofounder of Storytellers, a behavioral change communication consulting firm based in India. She is a behavioral change communication expert and focuses work on developmental and social change issues. An amateur artist and storyteller, she enjoys observing how trends and norms shift over time. Her interest in the subject of uric acid comes from a deep study on the issue, because many people in her inner circle have suffered from uric acid-related health problems.

Urvashi believes that seeing changes in our body and its functions can be scary, and we often want to stay in a state of denial. There is a certain comfort in not knowing what is happening within us. This book will help shake up that denial and encourage those with uric acid-related problems to act.

Soumitra Sen cofounded Storytellers, a behavioral change communication consulting firm based in India, in a quest to create communication that can shift behavior. He is a qualified pharmacist in India and enjoys exploring scientific nuances. His pharmacist-like mind has driven him to understand many forms of treatment, both in allopathic and alternative medicine.

With the progression of life, he believes that alternate medicine and nutrition has many hidden solutions that cure and reverse health problems. His interest in the subject of uric acid comes from his own personal suffering and overcoming uric acid-related health issues. His personal journey to healing has required a combination of allopathy, alternate medicine, and dietary change.